PRAISE FOR THRIVING THROUGH CANCER

"You present a truly integrative approach that I don't think I have ever seen in any other work!"

"I have read your book and loved it. I think that it is very important work and provides a perspective that is missing from the healing community and from the medical community. You present a truly integrative approach that I don't think I have ever seen in any other work. I enjoyed the way it was written and how you shared your personal journey with bravery and honesty. I especially liked the chapter on discernment. I have to say that there were several times when you expressed things that I have felt or known. I used to say that you can't fix a broken leg with guided imagery alone, but the guided imagery could help it heal faster. I have already talked to several people about your book."

Stephanie Windle, Doctor of Nursing Practice, RN, CNE
Assistant Professor and Level 2 Coordinator
School of Nursing, San Francisco State University

"Melanie Roche has written a literate and moving story of her journey with cancer."

"Melanie Roche has written a literate and moving story of her journey with cancer. She has then used great intelligence and an exceptionally diverse and high level of education, combined with a relentlessly adventurous and inquisitive spirit to produce a blueprint that integrates clinical, spiritual, psychological and social opportunities together in a way that can make any of us feel that we can thrive, too. It is a rewarding book to read, and valuable to use in real life."

John L. Barstis, MD
Clinical Professor of Medicine (Emeritus),
Division of Hematology-Oncology
University of California, Los Angeles (UCLA)

"Melanie Roche draws on the latest research in genomics to help cancer patients chart their own personalized path of resilience."

Steve Cole, PhD
Director of the UCLA Social Genomics Core Laboratory
Professor of Medicine and Psychiatry
and Biobehavioral Sciences
UCLA School of Medicine

"Melanie Roche developed our energy healing program at Canyon Ranch Miami Beach. In my experience she has a remarkable talent for gently getting to the root of clients' issues and facilitating important shifts. She is an engaging presenter that makes graspable the challenging concepts of energy of the body."

Karen Koffler, MD
Medical Director, Canyon Ranch

"Melanie Roche's profound recounting of her journey with cancer reads like a novel and satisfies as a story. Yet her inclusion of medical information, commentary on the impact of cancer, and distillation of its spiritual implications make this more than just a book. It is like a friend who goes with you to your appointments, says the perfect thing at the perfect time, holds a vision of your healing and helps you negotiate the (overwhelming) medical terms and personal decisions. Thriving Through Cancer is sure to become indispensable to patients, doctors and family members as a source of guidance and inspiration."

Sheira Kahn, MA, MFT
Co-author of The Erasing ED Treatment Manual

"Working with Melanie cleared my aches and pains and helped me connect to my sense of purpose in life."

Richard Krieger, MD

THRIVING THROUGH CANCER

Tools and Practices to Feel Better
and Improve Your Quality of Life
During Cancer and Beyond
- An Integrative Method -

THRIVING
THROUGH
CANCER

*Tools and Practices to Feel Better
and Improve Your Quality of Life
During Cancer and Beyond*
- An Integrative Method -

MELANIE ROCHE

Thriving Through Cancer
Tools and Practices to Feel Better
and Improve Your Quality of Life
During Cancer and Beyond
- An Integrative Method -

Melanie Roche
Roche Healing Arts
1925 Century Park East, Suite 740
Watt Plaza
Los Angeles, CA 90067-2708
Melanie@MelanieRoche.com
310-913-7233

ISBN-10: 0-692-80290-8
ISBN-13: 978-0-692-80290-8
(RHA)

Library of Congress Control Number: 2016918206
RHA, Valencia, CA

Book cover design by James Roche
Book interior design by Jean Boles
jean.bolesbooks@gmail.com
https://www.upwork.com/fl/jeanboles

PERMISSIONS

To James, and my mother, my sister, and Jerry

CONTENTS

These pains you feel are messengers. Listen to them.

- Jalaluddin Rumi

Why do you want to shut out of your life any uneasiness, any misery, any depression, since after all you don't know what work these conditions are doing inside you? Why do you want to persecute yourself with the question of where all this is coming from and where it is going? Since you know, after all, that you are in the midst of transitions and you wished for nothing so much as to change. If there is anything unhealthy in your reactions, just bear in mind that sickness is the means by which an organism frees itself from what is alien; so one must simply help it to be sick, to have its whole sickness and to break out with it, since that is the way it gets better.

- Rainer Maria Rilke, *Letters to a Young Poet*

INTRODUCTION

--

WHY AND HOW TO USE THIS BOOK

INTRODUCTION

Everything can be taken from a man but one thing: the last of the human freedoms—to choose one's attitude in any given set of circumstances, to choose one's own way.

\- Viktor E. Frankl

If you're picking up this book, chances are you've either recently been diagnosed with cancer, and you're having all the feelings that rush in when you first hear the words, "You have cancer." Or you're going through cancer treatment, and you don't feel so well, and you want to feel better. Possibly you've finished treatment, and you want to regain your strength now that surgery, chemotherapy or radiation is finished.

Another possibility is that you're someone who works with people going through cancer and other life-threatening illnesses—that is, maybe you're a nurse or physician, a researcher, therapist or healer.

If you're feeling lousy, it may sound corny for me to say, "Welcome! Welcome to the club you never wanted to join." But, as someone living with cancer myself, and as a survivor who's been through several recurrences, I want to tell you that it's possible to have cancer, be in the throes of treatment, and feel quite well, in fact, to *thrive*, even as you endure every possible regimen.

So what do you need as you go through all this? I've learned it's essential to have specific tools that can be useful on every level of your being—physically, emotionally, mentally and, if you're open to it, spiritually. You need a way to assess how you really feel at any given moment, and then, based on what you perceive, you need tools that meet your needs, and help you feel better, help you feel well. This book teaches you exactly that—how

1

to sense and meet your needs so you can feel well even as you undergo treatment.

I developed the Thriving Through Cancer Method and wrote this book out of my passion to live fully—to not be reduced to being only a patient, to not have my life energy get compromised by cancer, to live as well as possible for as long as possible.

You can use this book, based on how it's organized, in a few different ways:

1. If you've recently been diagnosed, or you like hearing stories of people triumphing as they go through cancer, start at the beginning, where I share my story, a bit about how I'm a walking challenge to the dire statistics of the type of cancer I'm living with. (Fallopian tube cancer, often "lumped in" with ovarian cancer, is considered the deadliest gynecological malignancy.[1]) As I write, I've already outlived the statistics.

2. Part II explores the need for the Thriving Through Cancer Method. Far from just being about cancer, this section explores how, in our hectic, busy lives, it's very easy to lose contact with ourselves and each other. Then when you're suddenly faced with a diagnosis, and you need to make decisions about what you want for your care, it's often a new skill to track inside your energy field and consciousness (and I'll explain what I mean by these in that section of the book), so you can choose what you want with discernment, and communicate that to your healthcare team, as well as to your family and friends. Start in this section if you want to get a sense of the larger societal issues and why there's a need for this systematic method. I explore technology and global connection and disconnection, what it means to be a sensitive person, and how to be in touch with yourself and open to the world at the same time.

3. In Part III, I share with you the four assessment tools of the Thriving Through Cancer Method, so you can track your real needs. Based on what you sense, you then put together a personalized set of practices. You might think of these as a "menu" or "toolkit" of physical, emotional, mental and spiritual practices, where you choose the tools that best meet your needs based on what you learned doing the assessments. The practices are also detailed and taught in Part III. This is the heart of the method. You sense in to see how you are and what you need, and then you work the practices that best serve you. In your life, this means you create a flow: as you do the practices and start to feel better, then

you check in with yourself again via the assessments, and see which practices suit your *new* needs. So you can feel better and better; and beyond that, if you want, you can use your experience for your own development. The practices work synergistically, meaning, as you grow in *each* area of your life, your *whole* life evolves.

The epilogue discusses genetics and epigenetics and points to the possible future of medicine. First we look at new approaches to cancer treatment including immunotherapy, targeted treatments, genomic assessment and genomic medicine, CRISPR-Cas9 (clustered regularly interspaced short palindromic repeats—essentially, "cutting and pasting" genes), PARP inhibitors (poly ADP ribose polymerase inhibitors that kill "bad" cells while not harming "good" cells). Then we discuss research in epigenetics, and explore what I call the "consciousness of cells." We are in the midst of a biochemical revolution, and this excites me for the possibilities of transforming many of the various types of cancer into what we might consider "manageable disease," much like heart disease or diabetes. As we enter more fully into this new era of cancer treatments, it is likely going to be possible to live a long time, even while one has detectable cancer cells in one's body.

There is an appendix that includes the worksheets that accompany the four assessment tools and your menu of practices, plus ways to check how you're doing. If you want to print the worksheets so you can keep them in a binder or folder and track how you're improving over time, there's a "pretty" version on my website, which you can print out—they're at MelanieRoche.com.

A Few Vital Points:

1. How to Work with the TTC Method:

—You can work the assessments and practices by yourself, and that is very effective.

—You can also work them in a group—for example, a support group can read this book, do the assessments with and for each other, and work the TTC Method and practices together.

—If you're a nurse or therapist or oncologist, you can teach your patients the TTC Method, and it can deepen your partnership for their healing, as your patient will be able to track her needs and communicate them to you. You'll then be able to recommend or teach practices that will integrate with conventional treatment, and at the very least, likely improve your patient's quality of life. This may deepen or renew your sense of purpose in your work, as you learn to sense energetically inside yourself while listening with an embodiment that calls on all your senses. This may be a new way of listening for you and a new, deeper way of being heard by your patients. Your listening with this full, resonant presence helps facilitate them learning the skill of being able to track and communicate their true needs. If you have any twinges of burnout, this can restore you to a sense of commitment, curiosity, and wonder in your work. The specifics of how you'll experience this will become clear as you learn the four assessment skills in Part III.

—For teams of nurses or physicians in group practices or hospital settings, you can work the TTC Method together, and this can make your team coherent, and make work enjoyable such that each person's unique contribution is valued. I'm aware there can be a whole other book on the application of this method when no one is sick, and I aim to write that book next. But in the meantime, these skills can be key to embodied leadership and joyful teamwork.

1. The Thriving Through Cancer Method is integrative and complementary. That is, the TTC Method is meant to serve as a complement to conventional approaches (such as surgery, chemotherapy, and radiotherapy). The contents of this book cannot replace a physician's opinion. It is not intended to be used to make a diagnosis or to recommend a treatment. To be clear: It does not and cannot cure cancer or any life-threatening illness.

2. Discernment is essential, and is neglected in so many alternative protocols and sometimes, though in other ways, in conventional medical approaches as well. I've learned the hard way, and in many situations, just how challenging it is to be in the unknown, facing difficult life or death choices. "Challenging" is a polite way of saying it; it's not an overstatement to say being in the unknown is often more than most of us can bear. It becomes so tempting in those moments to make decisions based on what we believe or what we want to believe, what our values tell us must be true, what we hope for, what we fear. We need a way to ask the right questions, and one of the most important, but often ignored questions we forget to ask when we're scared is, "Does this treatment actually work?" I explore discernment in great detail as its own chapter

under the section of mental practices in Part III, and I share with you a way to ask, for yourself, the questions that matter.

A Bit About Me:

Before I was a cancer survivor, before I was a cancer patient who has gone through five cancer surgeries to date, as well as chemotherapy and radiotherapy, before all that, I was an energy healer in private practice in Miami, Los Angeles and Amsterdam, and before that a medical writer in New York. And before that, I had a prior career as a choreographer, dancer and performer in New York. As a healer, I served on the Faculty of the Barbara Brennan School of Healing in both Miami and Tokyo, and worked directly with the founder of that energy healing modality, former NASA-physicist, Barbara Brennan. Her eponymous school is the only training program where one can earn a Bachelor of Science degree in energy healing.

Along with Karen Koffler, MD, and other holistic practitioners, I was invited to inaugurate the Integrative Health and Wellness Program at Canyon Ranch Miami Beach, the premier mind-body health resort, which attracts guests seeking a healthy lifestyle through comprehensive integration between medicine and healing.

I coordinated an after-school program for high school students who plan to become physicians at New York University School of Medicine. Besides my becoming a certified graduate after eight years of training at the Barbara Brennan School of Healing, I also hold a BA in comparative religion from Columbia University and an MA in experimental theatre from New York University.

The Thriving Through Cancer Method is a synthesis of all my mind-body training and experience. I developed it using elements from energy healing, body-oriented and transpersonal psychotherapy, yoga, meditation, my theatre and dance training, creative writing, my work with doctors, researchers, students and patients at New York University School of Medicine, along with my own experience working with cancer, first as a healer, then as a patient.

I have taught the tools of the TTC Method to some 375 nurses who are also practitioners of Healing Touch, another energy healing modality. I lead workshops internationally at such places as Kripalu Center for Yoga and

Health, the largest yoga retreat center in North America, and I feel excited to now share the Method with you.

As you can hear from my background, I've always been a "bridge person," passionate about increasing conversation between conventional medicine and complementary modalities. Yet I am wary of simply sharing anecdotal evidence of "merely" my own personal experience. I have great respect for science. So this book is partly a call for more dialogue. And it is definitely a call for research, a call for studies to see if this method, with its accompanying practices, is efficacious. To be clear: I would love to see studies that measure and track in patients whether utilizing the Thriving Through Cancer Method with its assessments and practices increases progression-free survival, overall survival or even "only" quality of life.

We live in a time when many disparate points of view are all available online, and consumer-patients are actively seeking alternatives to conventional treatment. The dialogue between allopathic medicine and complementary modalities is growing, but there is still often a sense of closed-mindedness, overwhelm on both sides at different perspectives, vocabularies, ideas of clinical success, and ways of measuring outcomes. We are all human, and there is only so much "bandwidth" we have for learning new points of view, yet too often there is a commitment to only one either/or perspective (either medical or alternative). This serves no one, yet as a healer, I know what it's like to wear "rose-colored glasses," and, at least initially, to draw conclusions based purely on belief, especially when the values that led to those beliefs dictate actions that seem sensible, not simply assumptions. So part of this story is how I grew from being a healer with confidence in certain ideas based on my training, experiences, and values to an expert in mind-body connection as a way to complement the conventional care protocol that evidence helped me choose.

At the same time, this is also the story of doctors' increasing awareness, based on research, that such mind-body connection is a crucial piece of the puzzle in care of patients with life-threatening illnesses such as cancer.

Today, it is with some fear that I share my experience of going through cancer and this Method (and I fear condemnation by the anti-medical people within the healing communities, as well as from the medical world). Yet I have been welcomed by the researchers, surgeons, and oncologists I have interviewed, as well as by the discerning healers who are interested in what is efficacious, so I offer this work as one voice among a growing mind-body integrated worldwide community.

I am not interested in having you become a "clone" of me—that would feel too narcissistic. Just as I aim to have you use discernment in all the decisions you make about your care, so, too, I want you to practice discernment with the tools of this method. Learn the assessments, choose your practices, and then generate your own. Use what works for you.

I dream of integration. I dream of using everything that works. I hope that by my sharing this method and practices with you, you'll be able to track inside yourself, come to know yourself well, moment by moment, and live your life fully and deeply. More than anything, it's my vision that your life will be meaningful to you, and that you'll have the freedom and time to create your life the way you want. I hope that by sharing my story and using my story to illustrate the practices, you'll be able to see yourself in my experience, avoid the mistakes I made, and shortcut your way to benefit from what I learned. Obviously, I hope we find a cure for cancer. But if cancer exists, I hope in the future the tools in this book will be common knowledge, so that if one has to go through cancer, it will be possible to do so and to thrive at the same time.

PROLOGUE

--

"CANCER RUNS IN OUR FAMILY"

PROLOGUE

Passing stranger! you do not know how longingly I look upon you,
You must be he I was seeking, or she I was seeking, (it comes to me
  as of a dream,)
I have somewhere surely lived a life of joy with you,
All is recall'd as we flit by each other, fluid, affectionate,
  chaste, matured,
You grew up with me, were a boy with me or a girl with me,
I ate with you and slept with you, your body has become not yours
  only nor left my body mine only,
You give me the pleasure of your eyes, face, flesh, as we pass, you
  take of my beard, breast, hands, in return,
I am not to speak to you, I am to think of you when I sit alone or
  wake at night alone,
I am to wait, I do not doubt I am to meet you again,
I am to see to it that I do not lose you.

- Walt Whitman, "To a Stranger"

In November, 1997, I found myself sitting on a small Formica bench built into the wooden stall of a cramped changing room. Wooden walls rose up on either side of the bench. There was a door in front, and my mom had squeezed herself onto the bench next to me. She held my hand. The changing room was in what was then called Beth Israel Ambulatory Care, on Union Square, in New York City. My mom and stepfather had flown in from Cincinnati just to be with me for what I was about to undergo—this brief, outpatient, excisional biopsy of a small lump in my left breast.

I had already said goodbye to them in the waiting room, and we said we'd see each other after the surgery. I had just changed out of my clothes and put on the scratchy, green, paper gown, yet here was my mom, wanting to be with me until the last possible moment before I was wheeled in for the procedure.

I looked down at her hand in mine. Her fingernails had ridges, the veins showed through her ruddy skin, and the back of her hand was freckled with age spots, but the shape of her hand, the contours of her fingernails looked like an older version of my hand. We each sat with our legs crossed, to narrow our hips to fit more easily onto the bench, and I noticed how we each kicked our top leg, forward and back, nervously, over and over again. Our thighs were the same length; we're about the same height, and I felt in that moment, like her daughter, yes, but also like just a younger version of her.

My mom, Nancy Klein, and my stepfather, Jerry Klein, had flown in from out of town because what if the lump I had found, that my doctor could not aspirate...what if it turned out to be cancer? My mother squeezed my hand hard.

As of 1997, she had been through cancer three times. She's now survived a fourth recurrence. At seventy-seven, she's had breast cancer three times, and ovarian cancer once. We joke that she is the only woman we know who's had breast cancer three times, when we only have two breasts. In her case, cancer started at age thirty-nine, and she was sick on and off for a decade.

Jerry, meanwhile, sat alone, anxious, in the waiting room. He had lost his first wife to breast cancer, and he married my mom when he was a young widower with three kids, and she was a young widow with my sister and me. This was not a story like *The Brady Bunch* though; no sooner did they get married, than my mom was first diagnosed with breast cancer. A devoted man whose nickname is "Wise Jerome," he stayed with her, and he's also alive and well at age eighty-three.

But not only had my mom been through cancer—the story of cancer in my family gets more intense: my father had died of renal cancer—cancer in one kidney that spread to his brain. He was sick from the time he was forty-three years old, when I was nine and my sister was six. He died when he was just fifty.

We didn't know at that point anything about genetics and genetic predisposition for certain cancers. We just knew "cancer runs in our family"—on both my mother and father's sides (and my stepfather's). My mom wanting to be with me until the very last moment felt partly like she was initiating me into a club I never wanted to join, and partly like she was just scared for me because she knew, from personal experience, all that's involved in trying to survive. The fact that she raised two kids, after losing her husband when she was only thirty-eight, and then, a year later, got sick herself—that amazes me. She's my hero.

Meanwhile, there I was, thirty-three years old and very healthy, or so I thought. I had spent the last several summers at various artist colonies as a choreographer- and playwright-in-residence. I had just finished graduate school the year before—I did a master's degree in experimental theatre at New York University, so I was always dancing, moving, practicing yoga, rehearsing, and performing. I taught acting as an adjunct professor at Mercer County Community College, and also worked full time as a secretary (with a master's degree! as well as that BA in comparative religion from Columbia University). I was part of the underclass of highly educated "starving artists" who make up the corporate and service-based workforce in New York City.

In my case, that meant I spent every day producing PowerPoint presentations at a big New York investment bank, about mergers and acquisitions of "new media" companies, and it was a very different world then compared to now: Not only did we not know about genetic testing for cancer, but the sequencing of the human genome (a massive project, whispered about with awe each step of the way by my colleagues at my former day job, at NYU School of Medicine)—while underway, did not show the draft results yet; and the complete sequence wouldn't be completed for another nearly six years. The blood test that could possibly detect ovarian cancer, the CA-125, hadn't been developed when my mom had gone through ovarian cancer, and the HE4 tumor marker blood test would only be approved as recently as 2008. The Internet was just beginning to be used by the general public, which meant mostly dial-up service. Researching your health condition online wasn't possible for most people, and there was far less content online then as compared to today even for those who did have Internet at home. The investment bankers I worked for were just beginning to have cell phones (not smartphones, but the old Motorola StarTAC clamshell phones), and these men (and they were all men, except for one woman), were ahead of the curve technologically: Email, photos, videos, apps, social media—these were not ubiquitous, and, mostly, did not yet exist. And though it's hard to remember life before all these ways to interact with other living beings bounced from small devices we hold in our hand up to satellites in space, and back down to other people's small devices that they, too, hold in the palm of their hand, smartphones were not yet available for general use.

Meanwhile, I was growing my career as a downtown performing artist in New York. The month before the breast biopsy, I had applied for a grant to make a site-specific piece in an old tenement on Hester Street. The performance would have been the same day as the surgery, and when the foundation's committee chose someone else, I realized that, had I been selected, I would've needed to back out. This marked the first time of many where my life has felt abbreviated by medical issues.

So cancer ran in my family, and I had lived with it as part of my parents' bodily reality from the time I was nine years old, and now there was the possibility that I might have cancer. But the news a few days later in the pathology report was excellent: the diagnosis was "apocrine change"—nothing more than a blocked sweat gland. I felt like I had gotten off scot-free.

At my check-up the following week, the surgeon told me about a study starting at Mount Sinai, in Upper Manhattan, of families with high rates of breast and ovarian cancer. She explained that the BRCA1 and BRCA2 genes had just been discovered a few years ago, and the year prior, in 1996, a test had been developed to screen for susceptibility to cancer based on these genetic mutations. Given that I was thirty-three, and that my mother had had both breast and ovarian cancer before menopause, my surgeon recommended I test.

I joined the study. A few blood vials later, and a conversation with the researcher when she drew the pedigree—the family tree of all the cancer among my mother, several aunts, my maternal grandfather, my father, his brother, their father—and that was all there was to it: I became an early adopter of genetic testing. I didn't know at that time how much of an early adopter I actually was by testing just a year after the test became available. I didn't know, for example, until writing this chapter, that those who tested had certain qualities, studied by researchers, and that many people decided not to test—they concluded they'd prefer not to know. [2]

What I do remember is when the genetic counselor gave me the results, they were hardly a surprise: I was found to have the mutation for BRCA1 at 5382insC. She told me I might want to think about prophylactic mastectomies and breast reconstruction along with prophylactic salpingo-oophorectomy. That mouthful of terms was more than I could take in. All I could hear at the time was "Cut off your breasts and cut out your ovaries," which seemed absolutely barbaric to me.

I scribbled the alternatives in my notebook, which seemed more palatable: We used the word "surveillance," which also had a different meaning then than it does now. I would get a mammogram every year, starting right away, much earlier than the recommendation then of age fifty for the general population of women. I would get pelvic sonograms with transvaginal color doppler once every six months. And twice a year I would also ask my doctor for that blood test, not covered by health insurance, that might indicate ovarian cancer—the CA-125 blood test. That I could do.

My resistance to doing the recommended prophylactic surgeries had a lot to do with my values (I ate a balanced, mostly vegetarian diet, never got sick, dealt with my feelings, expressed my anger when I felt angry, had good friends—all these factors that I had read about that I believed would protect me from cancer). And who was my model? My mom. She joined the same study, tested in Cincinnati, and—no surprise—was found to also have the same BRCA1 mutation. But she had had cancer several times and survived. I wanted to believe that, armed with this new knowledge of my genetic status, and my active "surveillance," if cancer started, we'd catch it early, and, just like my mom, I'd be fine.

There are a few other issues I didn't know as someone who tested so early, but now think about: In this time of rapid change, it's often easy to lose sight of how what people personally go through both gets affected by and has effects on larger societal concerns. Here's what I mean:

After that initial breast biopsy, there was scar tissue in my left breast, and every time I'd go for the mammogram, it would show. Sometimes when I examined my breasts, I'd feel the hard, tiny scar, and when the doctors did physical exams, they'd feel it, too. Because we now knew my genetic status, doctors would always want to biopsy the suspicious area. I had five breast biopsies of that same spot between 1997-2005. Fortunately, each time, it wasn't cancer. The problem was, I wanted my doctors to know I was at high risk, but at that time there was no protection for patients from health insurance companies discriminating against people with the BRCA mutations. The Health Insurance and Portability and Accountability Act (HIPAA) was just getting underway. As far as I knew, there was no protection against insurance companies considering any potential future breast or ovarian cancer as a "pre-existing condition," because the genetic status implied I was at high risk. I had learned from the genetic counselor to make sure my doctors never wrote in my chart "BRCA1," or "mutation," but right away, despite my asking a doctor to not write my status anywhere, in any documentation, even as he performed an aspiration biopsy in 1998, there it was a few days later, right at the top of my chart; you couldn't miss it. When I called to ask to have it removed and the record changed, the doctor said he couldn't amend my record, and besides, it was important for future doctors to know my status to give me the best care.

This was at NYU School of Medicine, and I had worked there in the past, so I knew people in that community, and I advocated to have my genetic status deleted from my health record.

The ethics committee met and discussed my case in May 1998. They decided to change my record and, going forward, to not reveal patients' genetic status. I felt relieved. In coming years, this became a more slippery issue though, as I became a self-employed person. Over the years, I lived in New York, Florida, and California, and bought health insurance policies in each state. Even without mentioning the genetic status, often insurance companies could infer I was at high risk, simply from phrases like "strong family history," or "mother breast cancer pre-menopausal," and the like.

While the US Congress soon voted to grant protection based on genetic status, coverage has remained an ongoing issue in my experience. As recently as 2014, when I was living in California, I received a letter from my health insurance carrier there that stated, "any future oral chemotherapy drugs that are available in clinical trials or may become available will not be covered under your plan." (And that was the only plan available for purchase in my ZIP code.) The translation was, the new PARP inhibitor drugs, the first of which, olaparib, was just then getting approved by the Food and Drug Administration, and known to be highly effective in those of us with the BRCA1 mutation, would not be covered in my case. At $13,500 per a month's supply of olaparib, if I still lived in the US and needed that drug, I would not be able to afford it. I'm sure I'm not alone. In the Netherlands, where I live now, it's one hundred percent covered.

So that's an example of what I mean by people's personal experience both affecting and being affected by the larger political, economic, historical, and ethical contexts.

Another example completely surprised me: After we tested, my mom and I together wrote a letter to our extended family to let them know our results, and encourage them to join the study. Given how many of my mom's cousins had had breast and/or ovarian cancer, and my maternal grandfather had died of esophageal cancer (the BRCA1 gene affects males with stomach, esophageal or colon cancer, usually in their seventies), we realized it was likely that others in my mom's generation and mine had the gene, too. We recommended either testing, or, if people didn't want to test, to at least do the routine recommended screenings every six months to a year.

Much to our surprise, some people in our extended family asked us not to share the information. My cousins were then newly married and just starting their families. My aunt and uncle, for example, said, "We want grandkids; please don't share this information." Years later, my uncle decided to test, and thankfully, he was negative. This meant that his kids—my cousins— were negative, too, which meant the grandkids are negative, so now there was no need for anyone else in his nuclear family to test.

My sister didn't want to test either. And when I said, "Honestly, knowing helps me. I just schedule my check-ups, put them in my calendar, and then don't worry about cancer," she decided to consider the possibility of testing. Eventually, some seven years later, she tested and was negative, too. So that's another example: all the years of worry, all the fear, all the discussion within our larger family—I imagine these issues come up in any family that tests or doesn't test, but where the members know or sense, "cancer runs in our family." As cultures and countries, how do we handle such questions? What frameworks do we develop for how to "hold" this information? How does the personal affect the political, and vice versa?

I interviewed several doctors for this book, and one of my surgeons, Richard Friedman, MD, said, "Melanie, make sure to include that you should have done the prophylactic surgeries. At least you can save other women from what you're going through." In 1997, I could not bring myself to have those surgeries (to prophylactically remove my breasts and ovaries), and I'm not sure I can save anyone from any "mistakes" they might make. But it's true that as someone who tested when genetic counseling was in its infancy, and with my mom as my model, I did not understand that if ovarian cancer or fallopian tube cancer (the kind I was diagnosed with) recurs, (and some say it recurs up to eighty-five percent of the time), that it is considered incurable, and virtually no one who recurs survives long-term.[3] Also, the surgeries have improved so much since 1997, that it's possible now to do the breast surgery as one procedure: you "go to sleep" and "wake up" with breasts that look like your own, with scars that don't show. The salpingo-oophorectomy can be done with the DaVinci robot now: the scars are tiny and recovery is quick, under a week for most women.

While I got great news with that first biopsy in 1997, fifteen years later, in 2012, I was diagnosed with fallopian tube cancer. One could argue that by not having the prophylactic surgeries, I "made my bed and now have to lie in it." But advances are happening so fast, with these targeted therapies, genomic medicine, PARP inhibitors, immunotherapy, and new under-standings of how emotions affect gene expression. When we lived in Los Angeles, Dr. John Barstis, my hematologist-oncologist at UCLA, used to say, "Let's keep you alive and strong so you can benefit from the new drugs that are coming." And I add to that, let's keep us all enjoying excellent quality of life, where we feel well even as we go through treatment.

Most people reading this book won't have a genetic predisposition to cancer.[4] But I offer my backstory here to illustrate how fast the world is changing in terms of medicine and technology, and to give you some context for all that follows. Essentially, by living with cancer in my family since I was nine years old, I've experienced all sides of it, all the roles—I've been the child who lost a parent at a young age, the child of another parent who went through several recurrences of cancer over a decade, and is now well. I've been the young adult who was well, but chose not to have children, in part because I did not want to die and have them suffer that loss that was so painful for me in losing my dad. I've been the single person dating who needed to reveal her genetic status, the in-love newlywed suddenly diagnosed, the person and wife who endures hair loss, hormonal changes, multiple surgeries—basically, treatment year in, year out—with a wonderful, patient husband who has to endure it along with me. I've been the teacher, healer, and writer who has big dreams that get affected by each recurrence—despite all this, still I maintain, you can have a wonderful life, no matter your role, no matter which stage of life you are in, no matter what you face. Wonder abounds, and you can choose to work with it, if you wish. The fact is, every living being is born, and every living creature dies. Knowing the truth of that reality can be heavy, or beautiful, or both, depending on how you "hold" it. While it seems it's human nature to deny or forget this crucial fact of our existence, the reality is, being alive means we are mortal. One possible way of holding this truth is to treat the knowledge as though it gives you profound freedom.

PART I

--

MY STORY AND WHAT I LEARNED BY GOING THROUGH CANCER AND RECURRENCES

CHAPTER ONE
MY STORY AND WHAT I LEARNED
BY GOING THROUGH CANCER

The cure for pain is in the pain.

- Jalaluddin Rumi

Keep walking, though there's no place to get to.
Don't try to see through the distances.
That's not for human beings. Move within,
But don't move the way fear makes you move.

- Jalaluddin Rumi

BC and AD

Ask anyone who's ever had cancer, and she will undoubtedly recall every detail of where she was, and what she was doing, thinking, and likely even wearing, the moment she heard the news. Like a huge historical event, like 9/11 for our generation, or the moment John F. Kennedy was assassinated for our parents, the moment you hear divides life into a "BC" (before cancer), and "AD" (after diagnosis).

I remember I was out riding my bike on a beautiful day in April 2012 when I got the call. My doctor called me herself. She never did that. It was always one of the assistants at the front desk who called. This time it was my doctor, and she was phoning me directly. Where I was precisely was under a

21

big Banyan tree on Sunset Island, one of the gorgeous Venetian Islands near where we then lived, in Miami Beach. When I heard my phone ring, I hopped off my bike and checked the caller ID. I began to shake when I heard my doctor's voice on the other line. "I don't know what's going on," she said, "but your CA-125 is off the charts!"

I think on some level I knew. I knew without knowing consciously. I had not noticed any of the conventional symptoms you sometimes hear about with fallopian tube or ovarian cancer: I had not had any pain, for example. Looking back, I can see in photographs that I was bloated. My round belly was big enough that it had made me look a little bit pregnant for a couple of years, but ovarian cancer didn't occur to me as the cause (even though, with the BRCA1 gene, I know I'm at high risk for both breast and ovarian cancer, so you'd think I would have thought of cancer as a possibility. But it didn't even occur to me). A woman at baggage claim at Dallas/Fort Worth airport, making conversation, had once asked me, "when are you due?" so I must have been very bloated, but I just didn't put two and two together. I felt great. Maybe a little tired. But I was commuting back and forth to Tokyo every six weeks, where I taught at the Barbara Brennan School of Healing. I taught at the Miami school as well as in Tokyo. In addition, I was working as a healer both at Canyon Ranch in Miami Beach and in my private practice. I was gaining weight slowly but surely, but figured that just had to do with being newly married: My husband, James, loves desserts, and I was partaking, often.

I did have one symptom that bothered me, which I hadn't been able to figure out: my urine had smelled for a couple of months.

It smelled sickly sweet, and I wondered secretly if I had diabetes. I had had adrenal fatigue for a couple of years, and I know that can sometimes give way to diabetes. That was why I had scheduled the check-up with my doctor.

She referred me to a gynecologic-oncologist, and in my memory, I saw him within just a few days.

When he examined me, he scrunched up his face and said, "I don't feel anything." And nothing had shown on imaging. Or, to be more accurate, nothing definitive had shown on the most recent pelvic ultrasound I had done just a few weeks prior. I did these sonograms twice a year as part of the surveillance I had chosen, because of having "the gene." As I mentioned, by having the appointments scheduled, I just didn't think about the risk very often.

During the ultrasound, I remember the technician, as always, would not tell me anything, but she called in her colleague. He looked at the screen and said, "That?! That's nothing. That's small bowel. See how it doesn't move?" I believe now she was right to be concerned; she was seeing the first visible indication of what ended up being transitional cell carcinoma of the fallopian tube, inside the open fimbrial end of the tube on my left side.

In any case, when I met the surgeon, and he didn't feel anything on physical exam, he said, "I don't think it's anything. And 164 isn't such a high number." (Normal is up to 21 on that version of the CA-125 tumor marker blood test, and I had never been above 15 or so in fifteen years of repeating that test every six months.) "High," he continued, grimacing again, is 800 or 3000."

"But you know what they say with BRCA1?" he continued. "You've got to get it out."

Again, I had known, but not known consciously what he meant. As he told me to go out to lunch, then come back to the emergency room, and pretend to have abdominal pain, where I'd then be admitted, and he'd squeeze me in for an emergency hysterectomy the next afternoon...as he said all that, I think unconsciously I knew what was in store for me. That morning, I had packed an overnight bag "just in case he wants me to stay," and I had made a list of other items I would need James to bring to the hospital if I didn't have that bag with me. I had left the bag at home, parked right in front of the table in our hallway where we dropped our bags and our mail each night. How had I "known," yet "not known," I was about to have a hysterectomy?

We went out to lunch overly hungry and in denial, but at the same time, somehow with the truth prickling at my conscious awareness. I remember calling my mom in Cincinnati and saying, "He doesn't think it's anything, but I'm going to have a hysterectomy tomorrow." Similarly, when James and I were holding each other the night before, I had pulled away from him for the first time ever, and had begun to cry. "Why are you crying?" he asked, as he hugged me. "Because everything's going to be different now," I said. Again, I knew without knowing, that I was likely in for a major ordeal.

The sense of unreality continued the next day at the hospital. Just as the doctor predicted, I was admitted through the emergency room. And yes, James and I sat on a gurney in a hallway in the hospital for hours, as so many do. Then I was sent to a room, and I remember that evening drinking bottle after bottle of the thick, salty magnesium citrate for the bowel prep. I remember talking with my friend Jessica on the phone the next afternoon when our call was interrupted, which made her anxious for me—it was time for the nurse to wash my abdomen and pelvis for surgery with the red-brown germ-killing Betadine solution.

Within an hour, when they wheeled me in for surgery, of course James walked with me as far as he was allowed. I went into a hyper-alert, controlling mode, where I was aware of everything happening around me: the movement of the nurses, the way one wheel of the gurney would get stuck as the man pushing it tried to turn a corner in the hall, the way my glasses were off, and I couldn't see anything clearly, but I was shaky and nervous. My body knew this was going to be a life-altering event.

Yet I was doing the surgery the "new way"—robotically. This is supposed to be an easier method for performing a hysterectomy: Just five little incisions, through which the instruments would be inserted into my pelvis laparoscopically. My uterus, fallopian tubes, ovaries and cervix would be cut out and removed through my vagina, which would then be "cuffed"— the tissue would be rolled over twice at the inner end where my cervix had been, and that inner end would be sewn closed.

When I woke up, I could press this button to self-administer morphine. I did a couple of times, but quickly realized I wanted to be as conscious as possible. I needed to stay awake.

I knew something was up the next morning when my surgeon came to see me as he made rounds. "Is it cancer?" of course I asked. Of course he answered that, "we don't know yet," that we had to wait for the pathology report.

Each morning he'd come check on me, and each morning I'd ask him more specific questions. "What color was the tissue?" I asked, since in the twenty-four hours since his last visit I had researched the meaning of different colors of tissue samples. "Let's just wait and see. Rest now and recover," was all he'd say. But he would not make eye contact with me. Somehow, again, though I didn't know consciously, I knew.

I share the details of my story because if you are in a situation where you are doubting yourself, or if you are thinking, "It's probably nothing, but I don't feel right," please do not ignore this feeling. Cancer symptoms can be faint. Ovarian cancer (which, as I mentioned, is what fallopian tube cancer gets "lumped in" with because it's rare compared to ovarian cancer), is nicknamed "The Silent Killer," and it is said to "whisper," meaning, if you have symptoms at all, they are often so subtle, it's easy to discount them as though they're nothing.

In my case, again, it was exactly like that: I had symptoms that were so seemingly minor, I didn't even consider it might be cancer, despite knowing my elevated risk. And never have I read anywhere in scholarly articles that the smell of urine is an indicator of cancer. Diabetes, yes, but cancer, no. A couple of women with cancer have posted on online bulletin boards about how they felt their sweat or urine smelled strange, but I didn't find those posts until after my own first surgery. But I was starting to search online for a couple of months before that initial doctor's appointment, as I tried to figure out what was causing my urine to have that sickly sweet smell.

So trust yourself. And yes, trust your doctors. You absolutely must find people you know you can put your confidence in to be part of your healthcare team. We'll talk more in the chapter on mental practices, below, about how to find and choose the right people for you to have on your healing team.

Some people say cancer or any life threatening illness is an "opportunity," a "chance to learn many things." That point of view always annoys me as being too pat, some platitude meant to comfort the person going through it, with absolutely no understanding of what it's really like. Yet in my case, I did need to learn some skills in life, and one of the skills I most needed to learn was to be inner-directed, to follow my "gut." These conversations with my first surgeon were my first taste of exactly how I'd need to learn to trust myself.

Then of course, a few days later, I learned that, in fact, I did have cancer. A half-centimeter spot, just inside my left fallopian tube, it had just spread to my left ovary and poked through the capsule surrounding that ovary. So, as we said, that was unusual—usually ovarian cancer, not fallopian tube cancer, is more common. And that transitional cell carcinoma--that made it a rare cell type. Normally this is the kind of cancer that happens in people who work with leather dye, or who smoke; it's often bladder cancer. I've never smoked or dyed leather. How had I gotten fallopian tube cancer? There is some thought lately that perhaps most ovarian cancers actually start in one or both fallopian tubes and then hop to one or both ovaries because they're anatomically nearby. But this is not definitively known at this point.

The good news in my case was that it was small. The bad news was that because my surgeon had not expected to find cancer, and hadn't been able to feel it on physical exam, and hadn't seen it inside my fallopian tube as he removed it, and it hadn't shown on the sonogram I had just done, he had not staged me. That is, the protocol normally followed to know how far the cancer has spread and where, so that treatment can be tailored to the patient, and so the patient has the greatest chance of survival—this was not done in my case.

Specifically, he did not remove any lymph nodes to check if cancer had spread to my lymphatic system. He didn't remove my peritoneum or omentum, that is, the lining of my abdomen around my organs and the sheet of fat that is covered by that lining—both areas where this kind of cancer tends to spread. He removed the fluid in my pelvis but simply threw it away; he should have sent it to cytology.

As a result, we guessed that the cancer wasn't very far along. But we don't really know if that is true. We'll never know. I was staged at pT2A, pNX--meaning, the tumor was stage two A, it extended from my fallopian tube to my ovary, and nodes were stage "X," meaning they weren't evaluated. There was no mention of the dreaded "M,"-metastasis, as nowhere else in my body was checked for cancer. The next further stages of cancer include cancer elsewhere in the pelvis, for example on the bowel or in the fluid in the pelvis, but as I said, mine wasn't checked. Nowhere "distant" (meaning far away from my pelvis) was checked either.

I did six rounds of Carbo-Taxol chemotherapy, currently the first line of chemo, meaning, the first combination of drugs generally used with ovarian and fallopian tube cancer, and I needed Neulasta injections starting with the second round to keep my white blood cell count high enough to continue the regimen.

Because of that lack of clarity from not being staged, after going through those six rounds of Carbo-Taxol, I said yes to second-look surgery in October 2012. Then, a lot of lymph nodes were removed from my pelvis and inguinal (groin) nodes, and part of my omentum was removed. What a relief it was to learn on waking up from that operation that it was "negative," meaning no further cancer was discovered.

That so-called "second-look surgery" isn't usually done anymore, as it doesn't prolong your survival. But I know myself. And I knew that because I hadn't been staged, I could not trust I was well unless I consented to that operation. As you can imagine, it made me feel ecstatic to hear that with fifteen lymph nodes removed, they were all negative for cancer. I was declared NED, "No Evidence of Disease." I see in photographs from around this time that I'm smiling with a dazed, exhausted, brave—but more than anything else, relieved—look on my face. My hair has sprouted back and it's short and salt-and-pepper colored--much grayer than I remembered it. But my eyes are crinkly with a smile, and I look like I've been through a rough ordeal but now can relax.

Where there is ruin, there is hope for a treasure.

- Jalaluddin Rumi

Remission? and Prophylactic Surgery

But my relief was short lived. After all that: the hysterectomy, six rounds of chemo, all the side effects—(from baldness, to chemo-induced anemia, to dizziness and breathlessness to the point where I sometimes would have to sit down as I brushed my teeth, and worse—if I was really dizzy, would sometimes have to crawl from the bathroom to the closet to get my clothes. I'd sit there on the floor to get dressed in the morning. After becoming so anemic that I couldn't catch my breath and had needed one blood transfusion, after hobbling around for a year and a half... [When my brain would say, "Walk," my feet would not always obey. I didn't have neuropathy; my feet weren't numb. But I was uncoordinated during and for a long time after those first six rounds of chemo.]) After all that, the toxicity that made everyday life challenging, and then the (thank God) negative second-look surgery, after every grueling experience that I—like so many others—went through, I quickly became terrified, pure and simple: Whereas during chemo my CA-125 had stabilized at 8, just three months after finishing chemo, it began to rise. First it was 9, then 12, then 16, etcetera, etcetera—in an endless progression up and up and up over the next year and half. During that time, I could not always stay serene or calm myself down consistently—as my marker kept rising, I knew what it meant: I was not well. I looked well, felt well, and seemed well, but I was not.

During that time, from October 2012 through May 2014, when I was officially NED, I also finally did prophylactic breast surgery. I knew having the BRCA1 gene predisposes me to both breast and ovarian cancer, and while I had been unwilling to consider what seemed like barbarically "cutting off my breasts" when I was thirty-three years old and single, now I was married and forty-eight years old. I was in a different phase of life, and the surgery had improved, too. Most important, now I had just survived life-threatening cancer. I never wanted to go through it again. More than anything, I wanted to live. Now I consciously chose to do the breast surgery that I had found impossible to consider seriously when I was younger.

So six months after that negative second-look surgery, I did prophylactic mastectomies and reconstruction to prevent a likely future breast cancer. I did the surgery in this new way, called "AlloDerm All-in-One." AlloDerm is a cellular matrix used to hold the breast implants in place. It allows the woman to not need expanders, and to do the reconstruction as one surgery. That means you go into surgery, keep your own skin and nipples, and wake up with breasts that look natural, like your own before the surgery. The only scars are hidden under each breast right above the inframammary fold (where each breast meets my ribcage). They are not visible at all from the front or sides. I am beyond grateful to Dr. Minas Chrysopoulo in San Antonio, Texas, who performed that surgery. I cannot say enough wonderful things about him. While that procedure marked the longest time I was under general anesthesia at about seven hours, it was the easiest recovery of any of the surgeries to date. Though that operation is also an example of how I had to surrender my biases.

A little context is important to mention here. At around the same time I did my breast surgery, Angelina Jolie also did prophylactic mastectomies and reconstruction, because she, too, has the BRCA1 mutation. She's since gone on to do prophylactic salpingo-oophorectomy surgery as well. She described her choice in an op-ed piece in the New York Times. That first piece ignited a national fire: It seemed everyone had an opinion about her surgery and, as a result, mine. As I considered doing the surgery and met with potential surgeons in Los Angeles, where we were then living, I had doctors say that the AlloDerm All-in-One procedure I was choosing, "couldn't be done." One doctor even went so far as to say, "The surgeon is just telling you what you want to hear. You're going to wind up with complications like the lymphedema you have in your legs now."

That was just cruel, as at that point, the lymphedema in my legs from having lymph nodes removed from my groin in the second-look surgery was making my daily life experience more than a little uncomfortable. To manage my swollen legs I wore the strongest strength of compression thigh-highs every day. They squeezed my legs with forty pounds of pressure. To get them on, I needed to wear rubber gloves, and it would take an extra fifteen minutes to get dressed in the morning just to put on my tights. It's not an understatement to say I hated them. I also felt they made me look chubby, as they were a thick layer under my jeans. They were hot and uncomfortable, but when I didn't wear them, my legs would swell, and that felt even worse. My legs would get so swollen and heavy with lymph it was an effort to walk. I've since found a way to easily manage my lymphedema with a practice I'll describe in the physical practices section below, but that doctor's insensitivity betrayed a lack of knowledge of my experience, showed he didn't know or didn't care about how to talk with patients, and demonstrated he was out of touch with the newest successful techniques for breast surgery, despite that being his specialty.

I let his arrogance affect me so much, however, that I questioned my choice of surgeon, the surgical technique I had said yes to, and even my willingness to travel for the surgery, to the point where I flew myself down to Texas for an in-person consult, in the only available appointment Dr. Chrysopoulo had before my already-scheduled surgery date a few months later. And I did this though he had already answered all my questions in an extensive phone consult, and I had been feeling very good about my choice before I met that other surgeon. When I arrived, Dr. Chrysopoulo said, in his British accent, "Good; I'm glad you've come." He explained, with great compassion, and by drawing pictures on a pad, exactly how he would do the surgery, and why there was no need for the expanders used in the traditional ways of doing breast reconstruction. He explained he would do the surgery in a way that looks natural. He explained how and why the scars would be just above my inframammary fold: This way, I could wear a bikini after if I wanted to, and if the bathing suit rode up a little, my scars wouldn't show. After being told by several doctors in LA it was "impossible," instead I'd end up looking like myself and, at least as far as current research shows, likely would reduce my risk of breast cancer to near zero.

People online and in conversations were trolling Angelina Jolie about her "barbaric" surgery. "How could she cut her breasts off?" "She had implants to begin with," etcetera, etcetera. Colleagues of my husband and even someone I had hired as a coach briefly right before I got sick all expressed their opinions online in their blog posts and newsletters. Their comments hurt me partly because I used to feel the same way: I have a stepsister who also has the BRCA mutation. (We're not genetically related through our parents; our parents got together and married after her mom died of breast cancer and my dad died of renal cancer. Though I find it interesting to consider that since we each have the BRCA mutation, we may be genetically related through some ancestor in the past.) Several years ago, when she opted to do prophylactic mastectomies and reconstructions and salpingo-oophorectomy, and I was in my "rose-colored glasses" stage of being a healer, I think I may have pitched to her "lifestyle modification" as a way to prevent cancer. She says I didn't, but in my memory, I think I said some pretty unhelpful remarks. No surprise that initially she didn't return my call when I tried to "support" her in making a decision about whether to do these surgeries as a young, single woman. And now I made the same decision. I did the surgery. I'm happy with how I look, and relieved I reduced my risk.

As my CA-125 kept increasing after the breast reconstruction, initially we thought it might be because of the inevitable inflammation that would have been the result of any surgery—that breast surgery, after all, was literally just a few months after the marker began to rise.

Looking back, those nineteen months of watching my CA-125 go up higher and higher were extremely challenging emotionally. That's a polite way of saying it. The truth is, I was a wreck. If the first time there was a sense of, "We caught it early. Your prognosis is excellent," by the time recurrence seemed inevitable, it was a very different story. Unlike when I naively did the genetic testing, by now I knew that once recurrence happens, and it happens around eighty-five percent of the time, cure is generally considered impossible, and treatment is only "palliative"—meaning it buys you some time, and then you die. I could hardly believe it. I was shocked and furious. This could not be happening! But I had done everything right! I had followed the brutal protocol. I had endured all those side effects. I had endured feeling awful for months. I had endured at that point, three surgeries, and now my old feelings rose up in me again, and I resented that I had "had to" voluntarily choose to "have my breasts cut off" and remade in order to survive. It seemed so unfair. I thought I was so healthy. I thought I could finally recover from cancer, regain my strength, feel better, and go on with my life. I felt like this simply could not be happening. And yet it was.

I'm dwelling on this because that time of watching my number increase and increase again, steadily, slowly but surely, with every test a little higher—that was the hardest time I've yet undergone, and it's an incredibly common experience. There were the endless visits to doctors, during which time they went from saying, "Oh, it's probably fine. Your number will probably come back down," to "You just did surgery. The number could be elevated because of inflammation," to "Well, it has doubled twice, so we usually expect recurrence, but nothing's showing and you feel fine, so we don't want to start you on more chemo; there's no survival advantage," to

"Yes, it's now doubled twice and doubled twice again, so if recurrence is going to come, it's going to come. There's nothing you can do. Look for it in three to five months." At month three there was nothing. At month five, still nothing. This "sword of Damocles" hanging over me was maddening.

Here's an example of how poorly I coped. I'm not raising this to blame myself, but to share how difficult it is to "be in the not knowing." As I mentioned, when the CA-125 tumor marker number doubles twice—that is, doubles and then doubles again, recurrence is generally three to five months away. The first time my number doubled, I was a mess emotionally. When it doubled the second time, I was so upset, I flew down to Texas again, this time for a second time to MD Anderson. I had gone there for a second opinion when I first learned I had cancer in 2012. And now I saw the pattern of the tumor marker increasing and knew recurrence was likely.

James and I returned to Houston. We met with the same doctor I had seen the first time, Pedro Ramirez, MD. He was the one who had said, "You caught it really early. Your prognosis is excellent." Now he said, "If recurrence is going to come, it's going to come. There's nothing you can do to prevent it." No specific diet, no supplements, no treatment would have any effect. I knew what that meant. I knew the statistics: What I was reading online at that point said one in ten women make it to five years.

I cried so hard in the hotel room the night after the appointment with Dr. Ramirez. I felt like he was sending me home to die. I felt so powerless. And I felt enraged!

My feelings for months were all over the place. We had moved to Los Angeles to be near James' family after I was declared NED (No Evidence of Disease). Exploring near our new home, I'd ride my bike, and be moved by the beauty of the desert around me. I delighted in riding my bike on a particular paseo, where every day I would inevitably see some rabbits. They lived in warrens deep underground on the edge of a drought-dry riverbed. I found I could be blissfully happy watching the nature all around, but then I'd burst into tears: "Am I dying? Will anyone even miss me? Why aren't my friends coming to see me? Why is everyone so busy?" I wanted them to let me know they love me. I wanted them to know I love them. I wanted my family and friends to accept me in all my rage and all my disappointment. It made me so angry when people would want me to be cheery or would seemingly get scared away because I was "too heavy."

I could not be "positive" or "upbeat." And it hurt when James would be so affected by my dour mood. It hurt a lot that he seemed to always want life to be light and entertaining, and, doing his best, he'd say, "No, you have to be authentic." But it was too painful for him to join me there.

At the same time, I knew and still know, he's a good man, and he was doing the best he could at that time. He didn't want to lose me. He kept "holding the positive," and I would sometimes get out of my own feelings enough to be grateful, and feel what he was feeling, sad at the possibility of me dying.

We had just gotten married three years before the first time I went through cancer. While I knew I had the gene and was predisposed to cancer (and had shared that information with him while we were dating), and while I had watched my parents go through cancer when I was a child and they were quite young, I knew that for James, coming from a family where no one close to him had ever died, and being with a wife who had been healthy and loving one day, and literally overnight was transformed into a very sad and angry person, must have been quite a lot to deal with as the months went on.

And my family—I got to learn so much about cultural difference. Now we can laugh about it, and it's even made us closer. But in that year and a half, it was just one painful conversation after the next: My mom and Jerry knew realistically what I was up against: the very real possibility that I would die "young" and soon, because both of them had lost their first spouse and other close relatives to cancer.

But James' experience in his family was completely different. His parents, John and Dee, and his brother, Mike, wife Gina and kids Deon and Jackie, are very loving people. They're very loving to me. I was very fortunate to marry into such a close family. John and Dee met when they were teenagers, and they're still very much in love. I call them Mom and Dad, and love them and feel loved by them. Yet they had never gone through a long time with someone going through cancer or a prolonged life-threatening disease that drags on and on.

So that year and a half was so hard! We had a clash of values. I felt that they kept asking me, both directly and through their attempts to make me "be positive," or "not dwell on it" to put on a mask of cheeriness. This was exhausting to me, and I kept falling into taking it personally. Rather than allowing them to have their feelings, instead I let their spoken and unspoken wish that I "be positive," make me furious. And I love them a lot, so it was confusing. Why would they want me to "fake it"?

I see now because the possibility of me dying brought up their sadness at the possibility of losing me yes, and also their own fears, their own feelings about dying, their own powerlessness. Again and again, I'd feel sad, angry or frightened and hear, "You're fine." "You look fine!" "But you look so healthy. I'm sure you'll be fine." Or worse, "You have to stay positive. Or death comes!" I see now that was how they showed their love for me. In a way, I was getting my wish; it just wasn't in the tone I wanted, so I couldn't hear it.

If you're rolling your eyes, or identifying with similar stories of your own, you can tell that cancer is a rough situation for everyone involved. And nowadays, it seems like more and more people are dealing with cancer or have already been through it. Nearly everyone knows someone who has had it, whether they survived or not. So how to handle the situation? All I knew was what I didn't want: I didn't want my birth family to say, based on their experiences and realistic perspective, "I think your situation is very dire," and I didn't want James' family to ask me to "stay positive" and "not dwell on it."

Sometimes it seemed there was no right thing to say. What I craved the most was for people to let me be right where I was, though I couldn't seem to give them the same courtesy. I wanted them to help me brainstorm "solutions," so at the very least, I could live as long as possible, and feel as well as I possibly could. Somehow my holding to that, and when I could, sharing with family and friends what I needed, has meant we've all improved at communicating our real feelings. We've grown closer as a result of being willing to struggle through these conversations. Now I feel we've been through a lot together. It's not what I would have wanted, for myself or for them, but I feel closer to everyone now. I did get my wish—I know they love me and now trust they know I love them: If we hadn't had to struggle through these issues, we might not have experienced the love so palpably.

The realization of one's own death is the point
at which one becomes adult.
- Lawrence Durrell, *Monsieur*

Recurrences

It turned out, the reports of my recurrence were not greatly exaggerated. My marker had increased from 8 during chemo in 2012 to 145 in May 2014.

We assumed we hadn't gotten all the cancer the first time. We understood—me and my ever-growing healthcare team—that we now needed to get as much cancer out as we could surgically, as that would be my only chance of having a proper remission. There was only one problem: we didn't know where the cancer was in my body.

Dr. Friedman, my new surgeon in Los Angeles, who I mentioned in the Prologue, informed me that unless we were very aggressive with surgery, I "didn't really have a fighting chance." A down-to-earth, warm-hearted, funny, very human man, he described the procedure: He'd cut me open with this huge incision, from my pubic bone all the way up to my xiphoid, right under my breasts. Then he'd "go fishing" to look for cancer throughout my pelvis and abdomen. I was about to consent to that surgery.

Then, suddenly, what hadn't shown for nineteen months on imaging suddenly showed: a solitary internal mammary lymph node "lit up" on high resolution CT. That meant I needed thoracic surgery, a different part of my body than Dr. Friedman's area of expertise in gynecologic oncology. I worked with Dr. Jay Lee, an outstanding thoracic surgeon at UCLA. That surgery was also laparoscopic, and this time we went in between my left ribs.

Dr. Lee tunneled from my left side all the way to my mediastinum in the center of my chest between my lungs. He removed the cancerous lymph node and some cells on my chest wall behind the node. This was my fourth surgery in two years, but because it was laparoscopic, too, the recovery wasn't so difficult.

After that operation, the news was not good: Somehow, some cancer had survived six rounds of chemo the first time and made its way all the way up to this one lymph node in my chest. This was the "distant metastasis" I had feared, and it was definitely far away from my pelvis where the cancer had been originally. It meant I was now considered a stage four cancer patient. There is no stage five.

The statistics broke my heart, and they confirmed what I used to fear when I'd cry as I rode my bike and looked at the rabbits: Now websites have been updated, and as of January 2014 there is new FIGO staging (so the improved statistics based on the new divisions of the various stages aren't available yet), but on the American Cancer Society website, it appears that according to studies of women between 2004 and 2010, the relative survival rates are forty percent of women survive stage four fallopian tube cancer five years, and seventeen percent of women with invasive epithelial ovarian cancer survive five years. You can hear how different these statistics are—

forty percent versus seventeen percent for five-year relative survival, with fallopian tube carcinoma now considered separate from ovarian. But the numbers used to be worse, with zero to six percent of women who would survive stage four fallopian tube cancer five years,[5] and one in ten women who would survive stage four ovarian cancer to five years.[6]

Still, one lymph node (doctors call it a "sanctuary") as a site of recurrence is rare, so I was happy to see my CA-125 immediately drop to 134 after that surgery, then 123, then 83. Normal is up to 21 on that version of the test, but the trend was downward, and apparently sometimes it takes a while to settle back in normal range. Dr. John Barstis, my new hematologist-oncologist at UCLA, said, and I agreed: it was safe to go to Europe for three months.

The summer was wonderful! I began to supervise students again, rebuilt my strength, and rode my bike all over Amsterdam. I taught a workshop at the end of the summer.

After that blissful time, back in LA, I returned for my checkup. The news completely surprised me: In those short three months, my CA-125 had more than doubled past the highest it had been so far—it was then 361, and another spot had appeared on imaging. This one seemed to be on the dome of my liver. I scheduled the operation and cut short a family trip so I could again do more surgery.

On the vacation, as you can imagine, I was more of a nervous wreck than ever before. And I began to have symptoms—my bathing suit felt too tight around the bottom of my ribs and abdomen. I felt a little nauseous.

Two weeks later, back in Los Angeles for the final pre-op appointments, I learned that during those two weeks away, my CA-125 had nearly doubled again: the morning before surgery, it was 660, far higher than ever before. That terrified me.

Dr. Friedman said, "You don't see a number like that without there being a substantial amount of cancer," so I was glad I had said yes to him this time going on that "fishing trip" of exploratory laparotomy and radical debulking he had originally wanted to do four months prior. Yet I was so scared. And honestly, not just of the cancer, which if I listened to those prior statistics, now truly was life-threatening, but of how I would look. I'm vain, and yes, I wanted to live. But I also felt like I didn't want a scar that ran up the whole length of "me"—from my pelvis all the way up my torso.

Dr. Friedman had introduced me to another patient of his, a woman named Claire, and she was willing to show me her scar. She smiled and was happy to be well, as she unzipped her gray jeans and lifted up her flowered blouse. She said, "Now, I had a couple of C-sections, too. But this is me." I admired her for treating it as no big deal. But for me, before the surgery, I was so sad about how I'd look with that huge scar. I cried and cried on the phone with my friend Béa. She comforted me. It helped to talk with her. But I was sadder about this surgery than all the others. I was sad for how hard I imagined recovery would be. I felt like my looking younger than my age, and how healthy I had always been was being stripped from me overnight.

I can't say this enough: Even though I had consented, and I knew it was necessary to hopefully keep me alive or at least buy me some time, it was still a struggle, and I cried over all I felt I was losing. I cried with James, I cried with my women friends; it felt like I couldn't stop crying. Somehow the hysterectomy had been easy, and I could "hide" the fact of it because the robotic way of doing the surgery meant the scars are so small. The prophylactic breast surgery and reconstruction caused more scars, but there, too, the incisions are hidden under my breasts. My hair that had fallen out from chemo had grown back, and while it was far curlier than it had been, I felt like I was finally looking fairly "normal," and by that I mean, not like a cancer patient.

And then this! I really struggled. And I can feel the sadness well up again as a tightening in my belly and a feeling that I want to cry as I type. Yet I wanted, and still want, more than anything, to live, or at least to give myself that "fighting chance" Dr. Friedman had explained: In countries where surgery is the most aggressive, he tells me that the survival rates are better. That surgery really is the only way to keep the cancer from growing beyond the ability of chemotherapy to keep it in check. And that since my first surgery had been incomplete, he'd make sure to remove any tissue, like the omentum, that normally gets removed in the initial staging operation.

So what I had most dreaded, and what I thought I could not stand, I did. Yes, I was cut all the way up the length of "me"—from my pelvis to my torso. And Dr. Friedman went looking for cancer.

He says that he works by touch as much as by eye. He can feel with his fingers little granules of cancer cells. That level of focus sounded and still feels most promising to me. When I interviewed him for this book, I asked how he became a gynecologic oncologist. He said that during his internship, when the students did their rotations of all the specialties, he saw how surgeons worked and thought he could do better. That's exactly the kind of surgeon I want.

We all expected he'd find carcinomatosis: these little "Rice Krispies"-like tumors that tend to be scattered throughout the pelvis, which is how ovarian cancer often recurs. We expected that the little spot that showed on PET/CT on perhaps the dome of my liver a mere four months after the first recurrence up in my chest, would be the "tip of the iceberg." Dr. Friedman said he had only been wrong once before with one patient who had a rising CA-125. In her case, mesh from a prior bladder surgery caused her CA-125 to spike.

In my case, when he opened me up, what he found was not carcinomatosis. And the cancer that appeared in imaging to be on the dome of my liver, was, instead, on my diaphragm, a much better prognosis. It was small, 1 to 1.5 centimeters at the reflection of the diaphragm peritoneum onto my liver. Dr. Friedman was as thorough as he promised: he removed my peritoneum, falciform ligament, ten aortic lymph nodes, the rest of my omentum, and my appendix, because it looked "scarred." The only tumor present was on my diaphragm. When I asked him why the cancer recurred there, he said, "Lie down." I must have looked at him with a confused look on my face, because he said, "Think about it. When your body is in a horizontal position, like when you're sleeping, any cancer cells will naturally go there."

I woke up after the surgery to the excellent news that there wasn't much cancer, and it had been in a tumor form, that could be removed, not the "Rice Krispies"-like carcinomatosis that occur throughout the pelvis such that it's impossible to remove every, single spot. Carcinomatosis is common with ovarian cancer, so the fact that what I had could be—and was—removed was wonderfully unexpected.

Yet, this was a hard recovery. The incision was long. Four days later, another surgeon put in my Port-a-Cath. Again I was under general anesthesia, and this time woke up to what I most dreaded and had avoided the first time I did chemo, a port implanted under my skin, just below my left collarbone. It has a short tube that goes into my subclavian vein, and from there into the right atrium of my heart. This port is how I've received chemo every time since, and while it took several months for me to grow comfortable with it and be able to sleep on my left side again, I have adjusted to it.

Dr. Raymond Schaerf, the surgeon who put in my port, is a cancer survivor himself, and he was willing to work with me and my "vanity": he allowed me to draw lines on my skin with a marker where the straps of my tank top would cover the bump of the port under my skin and the incision scar. This was and remains important to me: I didn't want to telegraph to everyone, "I have cancer," as I live my life. I didn't want to be reminded of being sick constantly every time I look in a mirror. My veins were small to begin with, and they were wrecked by my doing chemo directly into them during my initial treatment in 2012. Towards the end of those six rounds, my veins were so "shot" that it would take several "sticks" to find one functional enough even for the monthly blood tests. So I knew I needed the port, but I didn't want to be constantly reminded of its presence inside my body.

That was the second recurrence. After that I started Doxil, and between October 2014 and February 2016, I did thirteen rounds of it. Since Doxil generally causes heart toxicity once you reach a certain cumulative dose, and since my CA-125 immediately dropped back in normal range once I started, as time went on, we lowered the dose, then stretched out the interval between treatments, eventually extending it from once every four to every six, then seven, and finally every eight weeks in an attempt to stretch out how long I could safely use it.

All seemed to be going well; I felt great and was nearing the end of being able to safely use Doxil. Soon we would do a PET/CT and then go into watchful waiting. We expected I was in remission.

James and I had immigrated to the Netherlands a few months prior, and we were loving living in Amsterdam. We were looking forward to me finishing treatment and being well again. I had put together my new Dutch healthcare team, and we were very impressed by my new oncologist, Dr. Carolien Smorenburg, and by the Antoni van Leeuwenhoek hospital in Amsterdam.

All of a sudden at brunch one morning, my kidneys began to churn and hurt. I felt instantly exhausted. I thought I had the flu. James and I tried to go to a museum, but I was too drained to stand up all day. That's very unlike me. We went home, and I went to bed. A few days later, I still had a fever, so went to my primary care doctor. She tested my blood and urine and found I had all the symptoms of a kidney infection, but no bacteria in my urine. She sent me to my oncologist.

Dr. Smorenburg saw me that very afternoon. She examined me and agreed I likely had a kidney infection. She prescribed Cipro, but also asked me to keep the appointment for the PET/CT we had scheduled for the following week that we expected would show I was in remission. Much to our surprise, it unfortunately showed a 3.5 centimeter tumor on my left psoas muscle, along with a couple of "hot" paraaortic lymph nodes. We were all shocked. I had been feeling so well, and was excited to finally go off the

Doxil after a year and four months. But instead, likely by spreading out the low-dose Doxil to once every eight weeks, I had recurred, during chemo.

We immediately started me on Carboplatin again, this time combined with Cyclophosphamide. On the second round, I had an anaphylactic reaction to the Carboplatin. It's as though my body remembered that I had used it in 2012 and said, "No more of this!" As a result, we had to switch to Cisplatin and Cyclophosphamide, which is much more toxic for the kidneys, and requires fifteen hours of intravenous hydration before and fifteen hours of hydration after each round. This meant chemo went from being a few hours as an outpatient once every three weeks, to being inpatient, with me admitted to the hospital for three days of infusion every three weeks. I finished that course in June 2016. Initially surgery seemed like not a good idea, as the psoas is hard to operate on without potentially harming the ureter on that side. Yet the chemo shrank the tumor so it was no longer detectable, and the nodes after chemo were about one centimeter, so I did eighteen radiotherapy treatments in summer 2016 to clean up any microscopic cells. After that, we went into "watchful waiting," where we repeat blood work every month and soon will repeat imaging to see where I am three months after completing radiation.

As you can hear, I've been through a lot. While the statistics of recurrence and relative survival are dismal, I probably couldn't handle that knowledge, and so missed that in my reading as I went through cancer the first time. I had gone through conventional treatment, and it hadn't really worked—my tumor marker began to increase again three months after I finished chemo the first time. I had also tried alternatives—including wheatgrass juicing, a raw food diet, not eating sugar, particular supplements prescribed by a functional medicine doctor, intravenous vitamin C—and these hadn't worked either; none of these had had any effect on the actual cancer in my body or my rising CA-125. We'll talk about this more in the chapter on discernment.

If you're facing cancer, you're likely having some feelings as you read my story. The statistics are awful, it's true, but I'm still alive five years since being diagnosed, when that's relatively unusual. And throughout most of all this, I've felt well on every level. I have a full, wonderful life, and I'm grateful. I'll share with you what's working for me, and show you how to choose and use tools that can benefit how you feel, too. We'll explore this below, but first we'll examine the need for the Thriving Through Cancer Method. We'll consider the need from two perspectives: personal and global.

On the personal side, we'll discuss how your education and upbringing might have encouraged you to disconnect your mind and your body, and again I'll use my life story as an example, but now will ask you to reflect on your life, too (and we'll have a worksheet there, to facilitate that). In this chapter, I'll also share how I became a healer—which has everything to do with learning to unify your intellect and body, essentially, by paying attention to what you perceive with your senses, *which are in your body*. It turns out that the experiences that drew me to become a healer are more common than many people might expect, and I hear from participants in my workshops that many, many people have such experiences, and simply have no framework to discuss them, because these moments of perception fall outside the realm of intellectual knowledge. You can check if that's true for you as well. I also discuss how I changed and evolved as a healer: When I got sick, I went through a crisis of faith in my modality. The "rose-colored glasses" phase I mentioned-where I had so much confidence in what healing can offer? This all fell away.

Out of this period of intense doubt sprouted a whole new way to work with people, which I believe is more of a partnership with clients; no longer am I the "expert," where the client lies down on the massage table and essentially, in an unspoken way, wants me to "fix" her as she longs to hear my perceptions about her state. That always felt to me disempowering of the client. Now it's much more of a dynamic where I ask open-ended questions to help the client sense energy in her own body, and together we work with what her own body reveals to her. This results in deeper self-knowledge, and often, clearing of long-standing symptoms. The changes she makes in her life are organically her own, and because of this, they are right for her. I'm just the one who facilitates her deeper connection with herself. This is a deeply satisfying way for me to work now.

The second perspective on why we need the Thriving Through Cancer Method is more societal or global. Here we'll discuss why, in our busy lives, we are simultaneously both more connected and less connected to ourselves and our fellow living beings than at any other time in history. We'll look at what this means for how we "run" our energy, and how we can learn to track how we feel in the midst of our busy lives, whenever we want, on every level—literally "on our feet." This segues into the chapters that follow, where you'll learn the assessment tools and the practices.

If the chapters so far have been all about my "story," all about the "who," now we'll look at the "why"—why is there a need for a method that can teach you how to be in deep contact with yourself as you go through cancer or any life-threatening illness? What makes being in touch with yourself not already obvious, but instead perhaps a new skill? What can being in touch with how you feel, moment by moment, offer you, whether you're undergoing cancer, or you're the nurse, doctor or therapist?

If you're having a rough time, hopefully you can hear that I've been there—of course physically, but emotionally and spiritually, too. Hopefully my experience will save you time and energy so even in the midst of treatment, or, if you're a practitioner, even in the midst of a busy, clinical day, you'll be able to feel great (in all the senses of that word), too.

PART II

--

THE NEED FOR THE THRIVING THROUGH CANCER METHOD

CHAPTER TWO
THE NEED FOR THE THRIVING THROUGH CANCER METHOD FROM A PERSONAL PERSPECTIVE

Before you know what kindness really is
you must lose things,
feel the future dissolve in a moment
like salt in a weakened broth.
What you held in your hand,
what you counted and carefully saved,
all this must go so you know
how desolate the landscape can be
between the regions of kindness.
How you ride and ride
thinking the bus will never stop,
the passengers eating maize and chicken
will stare out the window forever.

Before you learn the tender gravity of kindness
you must travel where the Indian in a white poncho
lies dead by the side of the road.
You must see how this could be you,
how he too was someone
who journeyed through the night with plans
and the simple breath that kept him alive.

Before you know kindness as the deepest thing inside,
you must know sorrow as the other deepest thing.

You must wake up with sorrow.
You must speak to it till your voice
catches the thread of all sorrows
and you see the size of the cloth.
Then it is only kindness that makes sense anymore,
only kindness that ties your shoes
and sends you out into the day to gaze at bread,
only kindness that raises its head
from the crowd of the world to say
It is I you have been looking for,
and then goes with you everywhere
like a shadow or a friend.

- Naomi Shihab Nye, "Kindness"

Imagine for a moment that you are newly diagnosed with cancer, and you need to make decisions about your care. It's natural to feel anxious, and also pressured to make decisions. It's very common to feel impatient, as in "Just get this thing out of me!"

But how do you choose the details of your care when there is much to learn quickly, and you probably have many questions. For example, you may not know:

1. How much time can you take safely (to research, to get a second opinion, for example), without running the risk the cancer might metastasize or grow so much it becomes untreatable? Different cancers have different patterns of spread. If you have thyroid cancer, you have some time to consider different options; if you have ovarian cancer, you need to decide in a hurry.[7]

2. What are the different options for treatment? What benefit does each one give you? What potential consequences might each have?

Take, for example, the recent recurrence on my psoas muscle. In the back of my mind, I heard Dr. Friedman's voice saying, "Surgery is the only way to keep cancer in check; in countries where surgery is practiced aggressively, survival rates are better." Remembering that, I came into the discussion set on surgery; the pushy energy inside me felt like I was ready to beg for it. But when I met with Dr. Smorenburg (my new Dutch oncologist), she said,

"Surgery on the psoas is difficult; it's so near the ureter." I knew I didn't want a urostomy bag to collect my urine, and the thought of not being able to ride my bicycle or lift my leg and walk were both deal breakers for me. So, no surgery this time. Much to my surprise, as I mentioned, the chemo got rid of the tumor such that there was no longer any evidence of disease. The radiation to clean up any microscopic cells was worth it to me, especially when Dr. Wouter Vogel, my Dutch radiation oncologist, said, "Radiotherapy can give you about a ninety percent chance cancer won't recur on your psoas. Without it, you've got about a fifty-fifty chance it will grow back there." That sold me.

So you may find yourself making decisions for your care that surprise you, as this one did me.

The key here is to know what's important to you. Fortunately or unfortunately, learning you have cancer is a crash course in getting to know yourself well in just these kinds of very specific ways. And I know for me and for so many of my clients and students, nothing in life up until this moment prepares most of us to know ourselves that well.

What do I mean by this? You may say you believe "an unexamined life is not worth living," as Socrates said, but most of us mean it romantically, naively. When the stakes are high and you're actually faced with your own possible death, how do you find what you want?

A clue is to listen to and trust the signals your body provides. But how do you do that when nothing in our contemporary lives teaches us *to* pay attention or *how to* pay attention to these signals? Why is this so difficult for us? We're so good at other skills; our brains are so advanced, our technology so sophisticated. Why is this not an obvious aptitude? At least part of the answer lies in the history of the mind-body split.

Body-oriented psychotherapist Susan Aposhyan has written extensively on the separation between our minds and our bodies. She explains that Descartes was the first, in the seventeenth century, to describe mind-body dualism as a worldview. Before Descartes, humans were obsessed by our human capacity: As we learned to grow crops and domesticate animals, our sense of human dominion over nature grew. Technology and science increased that dominion further. Science arose and challenged religious institutions. Descartes lived from 1596-1650, and in his lifetime the battle between religion and science was growing, and, according to Aposhyan, both science and religion contributed to the fragmentation of body and mind.

After Descartes' life, industrialization reinforced this dualism between mind and body.

Aposhyan goes further and argues that the body-mind split had to do with domination of the natural world yes, but also of fellow human beings:

> "In the act of dominating, we forget our bodily connection with the *other*. In the act of being dominated, we become fragmented, losing touch with the vitality of our own subjectivity. The fragmentation increases cyclically; it is far easier to dominate a fragmented creature, be it human or animal or plant. We overlook the ensuing pain by moving ahead toward our newest ideas. We have become increasingly fascinated by our prefrontal lobe's ability to envision, plan, and create. Our fascination has led us to a narrow-minded pursuit of what is possible, what we *think* of, to the exclusion of what *feels* right to the rest of our bodily selves."

Aposhyan points out that though Descartes' ideas were popular, he did have a detractor in Spinoza, who argued that human functioning relies on both body and mind together, and he specifically argued that rationality depends on both the body and emotion.

She goes on to discuss the human brain, which she describes as being dependent on our hands and our tongue, and by extension, reliant on technology and language. Essentially, as we evolved, we created tools with our hands. These instruments allowed us to reach further in controlling nature, and both the reaching and the making of the tools stimulated our intellect, thereby causing our brains to evolve more. The more we reached with our devices, the more we could do, and the more we did, the more there was to talk about. The more we talked, the more curious we became, so the more we reached with our tools, which gave us more information to discuss, and the cycle continued. Our hand-eye coordination grew more and more precise. You have only to think about how we rely on our smartphones or electronic devices now to see this in action. Our fingers tap the screen and the tool of the Internet brings the whole world to us, right there in the palm of our hands. The more we expose ourselves to new ideas brought to us via our devices, the more there is to think about and discuss. The more we talk about, the more curious we become, and the cycle continues.

This is all fine and good, but ask anyone who's just stayed up late into the night researching about her life-threatening illness online and she may be able to tell you, bleary-eyed, what she learned, but she'll be hard pressed to tell you how she feels about it in her body: in other words, we live with the mind-body split all the time in our daily lives. And now when one is just diagnosed, suddenly the decisions are all-important.

So when we ask, "Why is there a need for the Thriving Through Cancer Method?" you can consider this separation as the root issue, and the healing of it, so we're unified and congruent, as the root solution. This mind-body reunification is the solution to improved quality of life (at the least), and possibly, if we believe the latest social genetics research, which we'll examine in more detail in Parts III and IV, increased rates of survival.

As I use my life as an example below, as I describe my intellectual (some might say hyper-intellectual) upbringing, see which parts resonate for you— was education valued in your family or not? Was or is there in your life a focus on the values of humanism? Do you "know things" with your mind, your emotions, or your senses, predominantly? In the US and in Western Europe, the experience of the split between mind and body is so common that we have phrases to describe ways to rectify it: "Mind-body medicine," or "integrative healthcare," or "complementary modalities." If the schism weren't an issue, we wouldn't need to specify the re-union or integration, it would just be assumed. As I use my upbringing as an example now, notice what sounds familiar in my story, and what feels different from your experience. After that, if you wish, turn to the worksheet in the Appendix entitled "Your Personal Life Experience" and reflect on your own life and how these issues may have shaped you.

CHAPTER THREE
BREADCRUMBS ON THE PATH HOME

For a moment she rediscovered the purpose of life. She was here on earth to grasp the meaning of its wild enchantment and to call each thing by its right name.

- Boris Pasternak, *Doctor Zhivago*

Breadcrumbs on the Path Home: How I Became Disembodied and Had to Find My Way Home

I grew up in a middle-class, assimilated Jewish home in Cincinnati, Ohio. The city is the headquarters of Reform Judaism, and, in 1970, my father became the rabbi at the oldest, most established congregation in the US west of the Allegheny Mountains. My mother worked as the executive director of various Jewish organizations in town. As compared to that heyday, the population has since decreased—today some fewer than 297,000 people live in the city, and particularly among the Jewish community, people constantly bump into friends. Our family was popular and loved. My younger sister and I were appreciated, and taught to value our intelligence. Our mental ability, in fact, was the most highly cherished attribute we possessed.

Our parents were both brilliant: My father was smart, educated, well-rounded, and assimilated. A second-generation son of German-Jewish immigrants from Berlin, his parents had settled in Philadelphia. Somehow in their process of assimilation into American society, they acquired a dream that one day their younger son would become—wait for it... (to our ears it must sound different than their aspirations)—an accountant. It was an act of rebellion on my dad's part to decide, after Temple University, to instead become a rabbi; his father had sold typewriters door-to-door.

The joke about my dad was that when he was chosen to be the rabbi at that most distinguished German-Jewish congregation, a synagogue called Rockdale Temple, that those on the hiring committee knew exactly what they were getting: Rabbi Harold Daniel Hahn was the only candidate who could also read a balance sheet. He guided his congregation to raise the funds needed to build an additional building. He was progressive, well-read, intellectual, funny. He knew leaders in the American and Israeli worlds of both politics and religion. A man who delighted in good food and the sensual experience of showering with Caswell-Massey cucumber soap, he dressed in Brooks Brothers suits and button-down shirts and ties, which he paired with Florsheim wing tip shoes. He did not wear a kippah, the head covering traditionally worn by Jewish men. Instead, he sported a comb over, with thick seventies salt and pepper sideburns, and the colors of his clothing reflected a businessman's version of identification with hippieish seventies style: Though he wore suits and ties, he favored sky blue, lightweight wool, pinstripe suits in summer, and in fall, when he'd swap the pastel suits for charcoal ones, he'd pair that corporate uniform with yellow button-down shirts and those wide ties with broad stripes in goldenrod and brown that were popular back then.

Currently seventy-seven-years old, and equally brilliant, my mom, Nancy Klein, is a Phi Beta Kappa graduate of Brandeis University, and she was the first woman in her family to attend college. She went on to do her MA degree in English literature at the University of Chicago, and then all her coursework towards a PhD in English literature at Wayne State University. She taught philosophy at the college level for several years. A Mensa scholar, she is an intellectual who believes in rational humanism as one of her core values.

Given how much my mom loves to read and take notes on a multitude of subjects, ranging from history to religion, and philosophy to art (as well as relaxing nowadays with a good murder mystery), when I think of the amount of time she spent teaching me how to spell, the endless cantillating of multiplication tables, I marvel at her generosity of spirit, her sheer patience, her ability to show her love by doing homework with her two children. With her presence, she gave us the skills that would set us up for life: my sister Barbara Hahn, PhD, is now a professor of history of technology.

As is true of so many assimilated German-Jewish households, there was much emphasis placed on culture: I studied ballet several times a week, and there were also weekly piano lessons, along with Hebrew school twice a week. We spent a lot of time playing outside in the afternoons; a generation ago, it was safe for children in the US to walk home alone from school. So I did, every day. And I savored that hour in nature as I carried my heavy canvas tote bag filled with books, always on my right shoulder, as I walked past houses plopped down in the middle of lawns that were each at least an acre.

I mention all of this because from a young age there was a sense of my body, and what my body could do, that was based on those long walks home from school, over the rolling hills of the Ohio Valley. My little girl legs had to work to climb those hills, and I loved the bumbling feeling of my legs being nearly pulled out from under me as I walked down the higher slopes. In the fall, my sister and I would slide down the enormous hill that made up our backyard, on "sleds" made of cardboard boxes that we flattened. The dry grass would get crushed and become slippery underneath us, as we'd slide from the top all the way down the hill of our backyard behind the house, and sometimes past the house down another hill that was our front yard, to the street. While this may not have been the safest activity, it was heavenly. We would also play hide-and-seek with the other kids in the neighborhood. That meant running across several of these acre-sized yards to hide. It meant skirting the barking dogs who lived outside, in the yards of certain neighbors' houses.

On Saturdays, my friend Tommy and I would carry a plastic bassinet down to the deep creeks that ran through parkland near our homes. The water was sometimes peaceful, other times raging. We called that bassinet our "boat," and there we'd sit all day, and paddle around in big circles with a long, narrow stick as our "oar." We'd hunt for fossils, and dig out clay from the creek walls. As you can hear, the rural suburbs of Cincinnati were an idyllic place in which to grow up in the seventies.

Yet even in the midst of all this play and physicality, was the sense of valuing the intellectual above all. But I had this other experience—the experience of feeling vibrantly alive in my body—because of my experiences playing outside. I knew what it was like to be "*in* my body," and that felt trustworthy, pleasurable, intimately intertwined with who I am. Though I didn't know the words "kinesthetic" or "proprioceptive," this awareness of sensing by how something feels in my body felt like home.

Between the two of them, my parents had thousands of books. And the books were not merely on display; mom and dad had actually read them. My mother's books were stored on shelves in our living room. Built in from floor to ceiling, the shelves covered three walls of the room.

My father's collection of books lived in his office at the temple where he was the rabbi. He similarly had books from floor to ceiling, and they covered three of the walls in his office just like my mom's collection did at home. His books would have covered the fourth wall, but that was a window. Still there wasn't enough room for all his books, so they were stacked on the floor in front of every bookcase. When this grew too messy, he had another floor to ceiling shelf built in front of one of the others. Double-sided, this gave more room for his collection.

So my parents were both highly intellectual. They were not what I would now call in healer-jargon "embodied." And I saw how my father's leadership was lonely: All his ability. All his talent. All his charisma. And I am not sure if it was him, or simply the leadership style of the time, but vulnerability was not valued.

What was valued was being a strong man that people could follow. What was valued was perfectionism. What was valued, both in our family as in so many Jewish families, as well as in the community, was being a "Good Person," capital "G," capital "P." The sense of "tikkun olam," the importance of literally, "repair" or "healing" of the world, was a formative value I inherited. This was and remains important to me.

I remember in elementary school I'd win awards for "citizenship," the concern I felt for fellow students. I cared deeply (and still do) whenever I would see someone hurt or bullied by their "friends" at school. Kindness was and remains an essential value for me.

But being a good person and concerned about kindness came to equal self-betrayal: I was too affected by what people thought of me; I wanted them to like me, and it bothered and confused me if I seemed to upset anyone. With friends, that meant I spent a lot of energy wanting to "fit in," to be "normal," to be loved. In my family, I felt like it was not acceptable to put any energy into or focus on activities I cared about, for example on ballet and modern dance, which seemed somehow "weird" or "trivial," because they didn't involve intellectual learning.

Especially with my father, I somehow got the message it was vital for my survival that I support him in his career. I clearly betrayed myself, and chose to spend my energy being the obedient, loving rabbi's daughter, rather than devoting myself to becoming a good ballet dancer, though I knew I loved to dance more than anything. I'd demonstrate my love by being exceptionally good; I was the stereotypical well-behaved rabbi's daughter or "preacher's kid." This self-betrayal was something I did without a second thought. My unconscious thinking went something like, "I've got plenty of energy to spare. It won't hurt me to put myself aside."

I also held the role of the "pretty" one in our family, whereas my sister was the "smart" one. Why we couldn't each be both remains a mystery, but it was as if we each took on our role, which was non-negotiable.

As the "pretty" one, not considered smart, that freed me to feel. This liberated me to sense connections and relationships, to be sensitive, and one might say hypervigilant to the nuances of energetic interactions between people, and between people and animals. I was and remain highly empathic. But this was not an ability anyone else around me overtly shared. I was often criticized for being too deeply feeling and told I was "too sensitive."

It was assumed that because I felt, because I was sensitive, because I could literally feel, in my own body, other people's pain, that therefore I was a bit of a dimwit. The overarching word for being this way did not yet exist, but I was labeled in my family a sensitive dreamer, and then when the term arose, "New Agey."

My rational mind was developing through my education, but it was only a small part of how I got my information. Still, I craved more than anything to be like everyone else; I felt a little crazy, and was only half-jokingly labeled such in my family.

And yet, there were always these experiences that perplexed and overwhelmed me which seemed to have nothing to do with what I was taught about how to process information. For example, I would dream vividly— usually bad events in which people got hurt, like fires or plane crashes—and then I would see images from what I had just dreamt as photographs in the morning newspaper.

If my sister or anyone else fell and skinned her knee, my knee would tingle, and I'd feel all the upset or embarrassment at whatever had caused the fall. If I saw a dog limping with one leg injured, I'd sense how the injury happened. Of course, there was no way to ask the dog if what I perceived was accurate or my imagination, and I was often told, "You make stuff up."

It drove me insane to feel like I could taste a strawberry, but I could never know if what I tasted was the same as what you tasted, even if we bit into the same strawberry.

At the same time, the rational world, the world of math class, say, seemed random to me. Why was the height of a desk 28.5 inches tall? How did we collectively decide that was the right number? I understood kinesthetically that making the tabletop a particular height was comfortable for the human body. But I did not understand why each one of those measures is a unit of measurement at all. Why was an inch an inch? The entire world of divisions of space equaling certain measurements seemed arbitrary to me. It incensed me that no one would talk about the why—why we had decided collectively that this amount of space equaled that measure. I wanted to comprehend the reason why, and when my teachers would throw up their hands, exasperated with me, instead of feeling that they were correct and I was wrong, I'd just shut down. I'd feel misunderstood, judged, not so smart. Stupid, in fact.

But stubborn. Unwilling to surrender what seemed so much more concrete. I felt ashamed, but dogged. I felt embarrassed, but tenacious. I felt misunderstood and dismissed, and, as a result, defensive and so dismissive.

As I grew older, I used my intelligence as a gateway. I transferred from Oberlin College to Columbia University, and I was one of only nineteen transfer students accepted out of several hundred applicants that year. Knowing how I felt dumb in my family, I did not even tell my mother I had applied until after I was accepted.

In college, I rediscovered my love of dance. I had studied ballet from age six until I was fifteen, when my dad died. Despite hearing and believing it wasn't a valuable use of my time or energy because it had nothing to do with the intellect, I had still studied ballet with a shrouded passion.

I danced so much in college that I unofficially earned a dance minor. I say "unofficially" because I was in the first class of women at Columbia University, and there was no minor in dance. Instead, I crossed the street and took class at Barnard (which had chosen to stay women-only, even as Columbia went co-ed).

At the end of college, I was faced with a monumental decision: continue on the path I had begun, the path of my family: to be an administrator of Jewish organizations, or choose to become a professional dancer in New York City.

My day-job during college had been to run an organization called the Jewish Women's Resource Center at the National Council of Jewish Women, New York Section. I had worked there a couple of years until I was promoted to being the acting director.

At the end of college, I was offered the position of executive director. I agonized over the decision. I called a good friend, David Sannella, a man who was then the accompanist in my dance classes at Barnard. I laid out the dilemma: Should I become the person I had been raised to be and follow a safe path of security, enough money, respect, the "love" of my family, continuing on in my dad's legacy? Should I honor the work my mother had done?

Or should I follow my heart's longing, and plunge into the wild, unpredictable, sexual, unknown world of downtown Manhattan, and become a professional dancer?

Like so many others, and like the stereotype of so many "preacher's kids," I chose to dance.

I studied at the Martha Graham School. I had picked Graham as her life's quest had been to find a movement vocabulary that expressed emotion through the body. Like any young acolyte, I wholeheartedly believed she had succeeded.

Every morning, I took class at her school, and after, I would walk from her studio, then on the Upper East Side, to Fifty-Third and Lexington to start the first of my jobs. I worked as a part-time secretary at a commercial real estate mortgage company. At night, after the office job, I worked as a waiter in a restaurant in the same neighborhood until four in the morning. This was a fifties-style diner where we'd dance to oldies music every few minutes while we bussed food up and down two flights of stairs. Then I'd get up and do it again the next day. (How I had that much energy, now seems hard to imagine.)

And while I could type fast and answer the phones with aplomb, I didn't understand the men who were my bosses in the corporate job. Their entire value system of putting on similar, drab-colored suits, riding the Metro-North commuter trains into the City from what seemed to me the great distance of Westchester and Connecticut, simply made no sense to me. These men were like the guys I had met at Columbia. I simply could not comprehend why anyone would choose to get married, have babies, move to the suburbs, work in the City, and commute back and forth by train every day. I couldn't identify with the desire for lots of money, the wish for stability, the longing to get married and have children; it just did not add up in my mind.

Like so many others, like so many generations in New York City, all that I lusted after, was the opposite: the wild, creative expression; the anonymity afforded by living so close together with many other people. People intrigued me. People different from me, including these executives, fascinated me.

Because I had the Ivy League education, I could "pass" in the corporate world. (An example of this was a friend's wedding in Greenwich, Connecticut. The bride was a friend of mine from college, so I put on a little black dress and enjoyed her wedding ceremony and party under a tent at the country club in Old Greenwich. I happened to bump into other friends of mine, all dressed in black and white, who asked, "Melanie, what are you doing here? Are you working tonight?" They were the temporary waitstaff hired by the catering company to serve hors d'oeuvres, drinks, and dinner.)

So I could "clean up nice," and then I could go back to "slumming," and spend time with my friends who were, as I was, making untamed performance art, and squatting warehouses all over the world to create one-night interactive performances. (We made performance events in empty warehouses in Williamsburg, Brooklyn; Dublin; and I made performances in Amsterdam, and travelled to meet people doing similar work in Berlin, too. Many of the neighborhoods where we transformed empty factories to host these all-night events have now been gentrified: The now hipper-than-thou Williamsburg is a direct outgrowth of those shows. [We moved into the neighborhood simply because the rent there was cheap in the late nineteen-eighties and early nineties. Developers followed.] In Berlin, a bombed-out department store in Alexanderplatz then with a restaurant, gallery and theatre attracted development money from the World Bank. In Amsterdam, a grain silo squatted by artists where I performed in the nineties is now prime real estate, one of the priciest Dutch condos.) That time in my life was paradise. I was broke financially, but rich in creative flow; it was heaven on earth.

I felt deeply connected to myself. Perhaps my career and lifestyle choice were mysterious to others, but I had a clear sense of my utopian nature, who I am, and what I cared about.

My dance training was proceeding. My body was strong and fit, toned and lithe and expressive. I felt everything. I felt it in my body. I felt it and sensed it among the masses of others in New York City.

The Walt Whitman poem "Crossing Brooklyn Ferry" says it best, and here I'll just cite two stanzas to illustrate exactly what I mean:

3

It avails not, neither time or place—distance avails not;
I am with you, you men and women of a generation, or ever so many
generations hence;
I project myself—also I return—I am with you, and know how it is.

Just as you feel when you look on the river and sky, so I felt;
Just as any of you is one of a living crowd, I was one of a crowd;
Just as you are refresh'd by the gladness of the river and the bright flow,
I was refresh'd;
Just as you stand and lean on the rail, yet hurry with the swift current, I
stood, yet was hurried;
Just as you look on the numberless masts of ships, and the thick-stem'd
pipes of steamboats, I look'd.

6

I too lived—Brooklyn, of ample hills, was mine;
I too walk'd the streets of Manhattan Island, and bathed in the waters
around it;
I too felt the curious abrupt questionings stir within me,
In the day, among crowds of people, sometimes they came upon me,
In my walks home late at night, or as I lay in my bed, they came upon me.

I too had been struck from the float forever held in solution;
I too had receiv'd identity by my Body;
That I was, I knew was of my body—and what I should be, I knew I
should be of my body.[8]

This feeling everything of my body and in my body, just as Whitman describes, was both liberating, blissful, and a lot to contain. It seemed like as I walked around the City or rode the subway, I felt through my body what other people were going through. I didn't know what that meant at that time. But it felt like I was a sponge, absorbing the physical, emotional, mental and spiritual states of everyone around me. Being sensitive this way was perhaps more to manage in New York City than elsewhere simply because there are so many people there.

As you can hear, I wanted to be free in the way that particularly New York seems to allow: completely anonymous, floating through the City disconnected from any attachments that might keep me tethered to any familiar role. Instead, I found the specificity of what I was perceiving more than I knew how to handle at that stage. I could smell when someone had diabetes; they gave off a sickly-sweet smell that I now recognize as ketones. I could sense who might have cancer by the gray cast to their skin and diminished energy. I could see who was in a difficult, perhaps violent situation at home by their posture, lack of eye contact, and what I later came to learn in healer-jargon is called "body armoring." At that stage, I had no way to confirm what I sensed, so I often thought, because that's what I had been told continually in childhood, that I must be "making it up," or "projecting" onto others. At that stage, I had internalized how I had been labelled, so I judged myself for having these experiences and felt I must be "crazy."

What did any of this have to do with dance? I didn't know.

But it wouldn't stop. It began to feel overwhelming because I did not yet have tools to manage this ability.

I see that I was using dance as a way into developing the ability to sense using my entire body as my instrument, as a way to know myself and others around me more deeply. This wasn't dance, nor was it dance therapy. I didn't know what it was. It was uncomfortable to be so deeply affected all the time. I didn't have a vocabulary for it.

As I've mentioned earlier, one of my day-jobs, when I was a dancer, was to work at the New York University School of Medicine. There I ran a program for "minority" high school students who planned to become physicians. In those days the aim was to train three thousand minority physicians and researchers by the year 2000, so the program was aptly named "3000 by 2000," and I was hired to direct the initiative at NYU's Medical School.

My first office was in Bellevue Hospital, a public city hospital, which treated poor, uninsured people, immigrants who did not yet speak English, and convicts from the New York City prison system. Many people came to Bellevue for emergency care as their only access to a doctor. It was not unusual to enter an oversized elevator and see a felon handcuffed to the railing of his gurney, along with maybe fifty other patients, from many other countries. There would be a few doctors in white lab coats in the elevator, too; we were all crowded in there together. I learned to not look away from all kinds of injuries to the human body, neither to look with judgment, but to stay as open as I possibly could to everyone around me.

I liked working there. But at the same time, I didn't fit in to the culture. While I'm curious about science, I'm ignorant and obviously had not gone to medical school. I found and still find the people who choose to become doctors and nurses heroic—especially in the US, willing to sacrifice their self-care to provide health care to others—but I found myself questioning the model: why did they need to work so hard and never sleep? Why were their schedules so grueling that they never had time to exercise or see friends other than those who chose the same specialty or worked in the same hospital? How did they manage to have romantic relationships? I wondered—when every time they'd put their hands on someone's body, I assumed they'd know the most personal details of what was going on with that person: For myself, as I learned anatomy, I couldn't help but recite the names of the bones of the skeleton as I kissed the man who was then my boyfriend.

Another umbrella term for how I didn't fit in, I would now label "holistic." The after-school program I coordinated followed the same model, the same way of learning as at Harvard Medical School: In one session the students would study a disease or ailment and learn all about that condition. The next week they would meet a patient who presented with that disease. The students would interview the patient not only about her or his experience of the disease, but about her or his life in general.

I loved that aspect of the program. But other pedagogical ideas confused me: these were high school students, and they'd study nutrition, and it was considered new and cutting edge at Harvard Medical School to focus on nutrition at all. I was surprised that no one had thought to instruct the students in the most basic skills of what is now called "nutrition literacy." So I added a module to teach them how to read and compare labels on food packaging so they could make their own choices about what to eat. I also asked them to notice how they felt physically and emotionally after they ate certain foods—candy, for example—and to begin to consciously use food to create the way they wanted to feel.

Similarly, my boss ran the cardiac rehab unit. At that time, I had recently discovered ashtanga yoga, and I practiced in a class several nights a week after work. I mentioned to my boss that recovering heart attack patients he was interested in teaching about "lifestyle" would likely benefit from learning how to practice yoga. Over time, after he reviewed the research, he added yoga to the program.

This job was a milestone for me as I got to interact with researchers, professors, and deans of the medical school, as well as the high school student participants, their parents, and sometimes the teachers in the students' regular schools. I felt like my contribution was valued.

I'm so grateful for my mentors there. I learned how to behave in a fast-paced, well-systematized, first-class teaching hospital, where decisions are made quickly and are often a matter of life and death, yet where it is understood that everyone is human, just doing the best one can.

Working in the "belly of the beast" of the American healthcare system though, also gave me an appreciation of how bureaucracy and cost-saving measures often serve to keep information from being shared across disciplines. For example, once, at St. Vincent's (a different hospital in New York, which no longer exists), I took my then-boyfriend to the emergency room because he had a high fever that wouldn't come down after several days. He was seen in the ER but sent home. A few days later, we returned as his fever still had not yet broken. He was admitted, and found to have malaria. He had been living in India the year prior, but had not come down with symptoms for all that time. After he was safely back home and recovering, I happened to go to St. Vincent's for an unrelated meeting with a colleague. I bumped into the ER resident who had seen my boyfriend the first time we went to the hospital. "How is he?" he asked. "He's okay now," I said. "But guess what he had? Malaria!"

The doctor had not heard. It struck me then that opportunities to teach new physicians were being lost, purely because there was no feedback loop built into the system to review the cases, and learn what happened to the patients they had seen. This strikes me as unfortunate, and a waste of the very resources the insurance companies say they want to save in their demands for more efficient appointments. More obviously, presumably if there were such a system, this physician would in the future recognize malaria, or at least have the training and wherewithal to take a detailed enough history that malaria would emerge as a possibility. Instead, that opportunity was lost. And everyone loses as a result: the doctor in his or her training, certainly the patient, the supplies and resources spent on two emergency room visits rather than one.

We will return to this issue of lack of feedback in the attempt to cut corners so as to increase profits, in the chapter on discernment below, because it is important in both medicine and in healing to have the means to confirm if what one senses as a practitioner is true, or based on assumptions that have no bearing on the actual situation at hand. Science is meant to test hypotheses and reproduce results; that's how we come to know what is true, and distinguish the truth from what is false. In research, this is straightforward. But clinically? The current climate of healthcare as a behemoth—particularly in the US since the rise of insurance companies becoming so focused on profit and cost-cutting—does not foster the doctor being able to spend enough time to take a detailed history, get to the root of the presenting complaint, order the appropriate tests, and then treat according to the results. In the various healing modalities the problem is often not even recognized as an issue, and there, too, this is worrisome: it's not unusual for a healer to sense aspects of the client's situation and assume what she senses must be accurate, rather than checking with the client, and, most importantly, rather than using scientific tests alongside taking the patient's history and giving the healing (for example, imaging, blood, or urine tests), to test the healer's "hypothesis." It's glaring, but not often discussed yet—but this is why integration is needed.

So here I was, this dancer, choreographer, and performer, working at a well-known medical school with its accompanying teaching hospital and with my office in a massive city hospital filled with the uninsured poor, non-English speaking immigrants, along with prisoners in handcuffs being wheeled to the psych. ward or prison floor in Bellevue. And as I mentioned, already supersensitive to begin with, my ability to perceive sickness in people was developing even more as I worked in these two connected hospitals.

I left my job at NYU School of Medicine to complete a graduate degree in the Experimental Theatre Wing at NYU. My aim was to become a professor of acting. To support myself during graduate school, I worked as a secretary, usually a "temp,"—those administrative and word-processing freelancers who float every week or day to a different job, depending on our academic schedule. I temped mostly at investment banks and big New York law firms. I finished graduate school the year prior, and was still working as a secretary by day, while teaching as an adjunct professor of acting in New Jersey at night and on the weekends, when I found that lump in my breast at age thirty-three.

CHAPTER FOUR
HOW I BECAME AN ENERGY HEALER

What is to give light must endure burning.

- Viktor E. Frankl

How I Became an Energy Healer

So there was that undeniable lump in my left breast, right at the same time that my sensitivity was becoming overwhelming to manage. In the Prologue, I described that first breast biopsy from a medical perspective, and in terms of learning that I had the BRCA1 gene. Yet that experience changed my life in another profound way, too: I discovered that there exists a whole realm of knowledge based on how I had always naturally kinesthetically observed and interacted with people. This marked the first time I had ever heard of energy healing.

The same week I learned I needed the biopsy, I happened to see a book called *Hands of Light* by Barbara Brennan on display at East West Books, then a mainstay of downtown New York City bookstores. I bought the book and her second one, *Light Emerging*.

I found I could not put these books down. Here were explanations of a worldview, a way of perceiving, that described precisely what I had always vaguely sensed. The definition and exploration of energy also corresponded to what I was then studying: In yoga class, I had heard the word "prana" (meaning life-force, breath or energy in Sanskrit), and I had felt the movement of prana through my body as I practiced the asanas, but never before had I heard energy described in a way that sounded plausible—that depicted us living beings as essentially composed of energy. It was a radical proposition, yet it also felt congruent to consider everything as energy. In this view, health is the flow of energy through the body, and dis-ease is the blockage of energy or depletion of energy. I could easily picture the analogy I later learned from Brennan at her eponymous school: She described energy as like a creek with water flowing through it. Energy naturally flows (just like water naturally flows), through the creek bed. Where a log has fallen into the creek, the log blocks the flow of water; it's the same with blocks in energy, each block impedes energy flow. Sometimes, during a drought, for example, there is little to no water in the creek bed. This is like a depletion of energy. Other times, such as during a flash flood, the water rushes in a torrent. This is like an overload of energy. By nature, as I said, the water gurgles along in a smooth flow. That's like when the energy is balanced, clear, and harmonious.

This conception explained why, when I saw heroin addicts in New York City, their skin looked flat, completely gray, with no radiance. I had not understood that I was seeing the way that heroin blocks, and therefore depletes, the energy field, but I knew how to recognize an addict who was on heroin versus one who was on another drug, say, cocaine, for example.

Similarly with schizophrenia, I had always observed that schizophrenics have a "bouncy" way of walking, where their heels generally don't touch the ground as they walk on the balls of their feet. I didn't understand what I was seeing, but I had always noticed it. Now I began to understand what being "ungrounded" and having one's energy field be "too permeable" might look like—"ungrounded" was not "new-agey," but rather a literal description.

Barbara Brennan had been a physicist at NASA, and her tone was a combination of scientific writing translated for laypeople, combined with this other—let's call it Eastern philosophical—material. Never before had I heard of a NASA physicist who could discuss the chakra system from Ayurveda (the Hindu system of medicine). Have you ever had an experience of reading a book where with every sentence you say to yourself, again and again,"Yes! Yes! That's exactly how it is." That's how I felt at that stage, reading Brennan's books.

And here I was, faced with surgery and the potential that this lump in my breast might be breast cancer. As I said, given that I had watched both my parents go through cancer, I did not want that to be my story.

A former dance mentor of mine in Cincinnati, Fanchon Shur, had graduated from the four years of training at the Barbara Brennan School of

Healing. I called Fanchon and asked her to refer me to a colleague in New York. She chose Joan MacIntosh.

I had heard of Joan. A well-known actor in the world of downtown New York experimental theatre, she had formerly been married to Richard Schechner, a theatre director and Chairman of performance studies at New York University. He had been my mentor in graduate school, and had published my first article about making theatre in empty warehouses, in the academic performance studies journal that he edits, *TDR/The Drama Review.*

My first energy healing appointment with Joan took place between the appointment with my doctor where she attempted the needle aspiration, and then the surgical appointment for the excisional biopsy. It's not an overstatement to say that healing changed my life.

Sitting on her couch in her office on the Upper West Side, I remember crying. I had written a play in graduate school and had gotten in a lot of trouble for it: I had nearly been expelled from the Experimental Theatre Wing at NYU. The play concerned the connection between two people who would ordinarily feel they had nothing in common—a homeless man and an upper middle class woman who has breast cancer. (You can tell the play was highly autobiographical.)

This play was all about how we humans choose to either energetically perceive the connections between people, or not—to sense what I call resonance. We'll explore resonance as one of the skills of the Thriving Through Cancer Method, and I'll share with you how you can resonate and perceive resonance, too. What I tried to delve into in that play was the possibility that we humans are as energetically connected with one another as we allow ourselves to be, and that we have a choice about sensing that much energetically. To make this more concrete, consider how you feel—in your body (that is, what your bodily response or reaction is)—when you click on a news story link and immediately a video begins to play that shows a fellow human being suffering, injured, or killed. Internet access was still new in 1995,[9] but already it felt like we were beginning to be bombarded by images of each other's experiences, along with the nonstop coverage of world events which have since become ubiquitous. And if we had the capacity for empathy, it seemed our encounters with others were developing that line of intelligence in us even more rapidly than in the recent past, before the Internet. So two people who feel they have nothing in common actually have similar concerns or fears. Specifically, in my play, the character of the homeless man feels he needs to have "a visible mark," a scar, so he looks like "a warrior, worthy of respect." Meanwhile, the middle-class woman feels she *has* a "visible mark" by virtue of having had mastectomies. She's worried "everyone will know" she's been through cancer. You can hear what I described earlier as my sensitivity growing; now I tried to put into dialogue all my feelings about what having such awareness evoked. I was clearly using my creative work as a way to resolve how to handle being affected by others; now I see this was leading towards my passion for healing.

But I didn't recognize any of that then. As I sat in Joan's office that day, she sat in a chair facing me; her Siamese cats climbed all over her as she listened. I cried about the play I had written, how it hadn't brought me the "big break" I had so longed for. It also hadn't gotten me any letters of recommendation from my teachers at NYU. On the contrary, it felt like by writing and producing the play I had "killed off" my ability to earn a living as a professor of theatre at any university.

I cried not only about the play, but about my disappointment in romantic relationships. I cried about the cancer in my family, and as you can imagine, given that history, I was just so frightened I might have cancer. I was so healthy and young, I just didn't think it was possible for me to be sick, but I was terrified.

I sat weeping on Joan's couch as I let these fears pour out of me, and she said, "Look down."

She had these crystals hanging in her windows, and the sunlight was shining through one of them; it made a rainbow on my shirt right where the lump was.

"This isn't about your play, " she said. "It isn't about the cancer in your family. This is about your creativity. And I guarantee you, if you stick with this process, you're going to get your creativity back."

I didn't know what she meant. But I liked the sound of it. And her voice was both direct and soothing at the same time.

We moved to the table work. Unlike in massage, I took my shoes off but was otherwise fully clothed. I lay down on my back on her massage table. She put her hands on my feet, and immediately I felt like I was being filled up with water, as though I was a pitcher, and warm water was flowing into me, filling up my entire body. I knew I had never before felt anything like this, and that I was not imagining it. It had a "whoosh, whoosh," sound, like it was pulsing into me. It felt comforting and energizing at the same time. But strange. It definitely piqued my curiosity.

After the healing, when I got up from the massage table, Joan said, "Don't get on the subway right away. You're going to feel a little weird. Go sit in the park." She meant Riverside Park, which was near her apartment. As I walked there, it was that hour when nannies push kids in strollers, so they'll be back home in time for their parents then on their way from work.

It was the oddest experience: One by one, as each stroller passed, every kid reached out her or his hands to me, as if to say, "Pick me up! Play with me!" Having no kids of my own, and always having felt awkward around children, this was remarkable.

Similarly, dogs on leashes were being walked past me, and each one would tug on the leash and run towards me, as if to say, "Let's play!" I had never experienced anything like this before in my life. One dog, maybe. But every dog, and every child? No.

When I got to Riverside Park, I longed to sit on the ground. If you know New York City, you know you never sit on the ground. But that was clearly what I wanted. I found a tree with not too much litter in the dust around the trunk, and I plopped my butt in the dirt. I looked down the hill, across the Hudson River to New Jersey, and the way the sunlight was glinting on the water, the way the wind was rustling the leaves in the branches above my head, I felt this sudden rush of understanding: "I get it!" I thought. "The world exists at a particular frequency, a certain tempo, a specific speed, and I'm back to being in alignment with that frequency or vibration." Having never recognized I was out of alignment before, I felt profoundly what it meant to be unified with this vibration.

So it's true, I'm a healer, and you might expect me to use words like "frequency" and "vibration." But I can assure you, this was not how I talked. Yet the experience was palpable, concrete, specific, and unique.

Two days later, I had that first breast biopsy that set the stage for my journey through genetic testing (and then, fifteen years later, through the first occurrence of cancer). And when, a few days later, the pathology report came back with the diagnosis of "apocrine change"—a blocked sweat gland—I was curious: How did the cells go from being "suspicious" in the initial aspiration, to merely a blocked sweat gland? Did that first healing "cure" a cancer that was starting in my body? At this point in time, we have no test, no means to assess whether cells are able to revert back to normal after they've run amok. We may never know with that tissue sample, but the apparent change made me want to know more. I began to work with Joan for healing sessions weekly.

And my life began to change. I left the secretarial job because I got hired to write a streaming video for the Internet. (This was during the dot-com bubble, and it marked the first time I had been hired to write professionally.) I had been dating a man who was fine, but not for me. I left that relationship, and began to go on dates with men where I showed more of myself in relationship. In other words, I began to take off my "mask"—all the ways I tried to fit in; instead I began to reveal more of who I really am.

About two years into my process of working with Joan, I had an unusual dream, unlike any I had ever had. In the dream, I was studying with a Native American teacher. My job was to take care of his two daughters and sweep up around the fireplace. One day, I took the daughters outside for a walk, and I saw a beautiful "something" in the sky. It was a kite, but not shaped like a kite; it was shaped more like a house, the two diagonal lines of the roof coming to a point at the apex, then the boxy, square shape of the house underneath. It was made of pulsing light, and it included all the colors of the rainbow. It had tails streaming from its base. There were pairs of them, and they were longer on the outer sides with each pair shorter, the closer they hung towards the center of the base. The outer, longest pairs were red, the next closer to the center were orange. The next were yellow, then green, then blue, then indigo, ending with one white tail in the center. This kite-that-resembled-a-house was in the sky, and it was the most beautiful "thing" I had ever seen.

In the dream, I crossed my hands over my chest, because I wanted it, and felt it was too much to long for. It was too beautiful, and somehow I felt like I shouldn't desire it; it wasn't meant for me; I couldn't allow myself to want it. It somehow telepathically communicated to me, "It's for you! Open your arms and receive it." I did.

When we got back to the house, my teacher was sweeping up around the fireplace, and he nonchalantly said, "Oh, congratulations. That's called an 'amochenko.' And you're supposed to wear it 'here'" (he indicated the front of a person's upper chest, above the breasts and lower than the throat), "and 'here,'" the same spot in back (essentially, between one's shoulder blades).

I didn't know it at the time, but in Barbara Brennan's conception of energy healing, that spot in front is called the "soul seat." It's where your longing for this lifetime is said to reside.

I was also told in the dream to go to healing school, and eventually to name my healing practice Amochenko Healing Arts, Inc. The idea was that no one would know what an "amochenko" is, and everyone would ask.

Because they would ask, I could share my story of how I came to change careers and become an energy healer.

I woke up that morning with the clear feeling, "I'm meant to be an energy healer. I'm going to find a way to attend the Barbara Brennan School of Healing."

It took me a year, but I did eventually start school. Despite already having that master's degree in theatre from New York University, and despite the BA in comparative religion from Columbia University, I jumped in completely to the training at BBSH.

From the first moments, I loved the material, and found it came easily to me. After completing the four years of the program, I became a certified graduate, then completed four more years in the advanced studies program (to learn to teach the work), and the Brennan Integration Program (which synthesizes energy healing with psychotherapeutic methods). This allows me to be a "BIP," a Brennan Integration Practitioner, and supervise students as they go through the training. I taught at the Barbara Brennan School of Healing for four years in Miami and a year in Tokyo, and left in 2010 to develop what has grown into this work. When I first got sick in 2012, I took everything I knew as a healer, dancer, choreographer, actor, director and writer, and applied it specifically to helping me live as well as possible as I went through cancer. I developed the Thriving Through Cancer Method as an integration of all I know.

In addition to teaching at the School, I also grew my private practice. When not sick with cancer, I work with students, but mostly work with people not connected with the School. These people come to me because they want the mind-body connection that I bring, and often they want energy healing specifically. I work with clients all over the world, by phone, by Skype and in person.

I love working this way, and enjoy my work very much. I've seen people go from being in constant physical pain, miserable in their work and personal lives, to being well, in great relationships, doing what they love to do. I've helped people in their marriages, in their businesses, the companies they've founded, the organizations they lead. I've helped people before, during, and after surgery. Typically my clients need less pain medication after surgery and recover faster than expected.[10] For example, one client, "P" had surgery for an umbilical hernia, and was expected to not be able to walk up stairs for several weeks. She was told to move her bed downstairs before the surgery, and that she'd be home from work for six weeks. Instead, she was off pain meds. within a week, could walk up stairs easily after a week and a half, and so had a vacation from work, during which time she felt well.

I've helped people with Parkinson's disease walk with less of a shuffling gait. I've helped people with back pain avoid surgery, even when they didn't "believe" in healing and were convinced they'd need the operation. "Oh my God, I feel something!" one of these clients said, in his Southern accent, as I put my hands on his feet the first time.

I've been honored to be part of a healing team, along with clients' psychiatrists, to help clients with bipolar disorder, gradually, safely, and with the psychiatrists' supervision and permission, reduce dosage of the medications such as Depakote taken to treat and manage bipolar disorder. I've worked as a complementary practitioner for patients undergoing chemotherapy. I've worked in hospitals, for example with a patient in the first days after liver transplant. I've been present with people as they die, and, at the same time, been there with family members during the time of their loved one dying.

These experiences have had a profound effect on my life.

I share these experiences to describe my initial process of how I integrated healing with conventional medicine. Nowadays, complementary and alternative modalities (CAM) are often known about, and many people utilize some form of CAM if they feel it can be beneficial. No matter whether you address your healthcare issues with solely allopathic medicine or some combination of CAM, you get to choose the qualities of your healthcare providers. And if you're the healthcare professional, you, too, get to choose: What qualities are important to you in the way that you practice medicine and/or healing?

As we turn our attention from my story to yours now, let's examine the qualities important in practitioners and in patients. There are two descriptions of qualities below. First is a list of qualities of being a practitioner. The second is a list of qualities of being a patient. After you read through the lists, turn the worksheet in the appendix, and, thinking about your own preferences, complete the worksheet. I believe that whether you're currently a patient or currently a healthcare professional, you can fill out the list for both roles.

For example, if you're the patient choosing the qualities you want in your healthcare team, obviously the description of qualities of a healthcare professional is relevant for you. But you also may wish to consider the qualities you bring as a patient, and make choices about how you want to be, which qualities you want to bring to your interactions with your doctors, nurses, healers, and other healthcare professionals, so that you can get the best care possible.

The same is true if you're a doctor, nurse, or healer in any modality: Obviously, it's relevant to consider the qualities you bring as a practitioner, but it's also likely useful to consider the qualities in patients or clients that help you feel you can do your best work. Consider this list a jumping off point, and then complete the worksheet in the appendix based on what you discover. Can you train your patients to bring the qualities you need so you can serve them in the best way possible? I believe you can, and that patients appreciate such guidance from you.

For me, the characteristics that I bring which I value as a practitioner mostly have to do with the ability to translate between different modalities and vocabularies, as well as to be as present as I can with clients. The sensitivity I've been describing throughout this part of the book? It's become the most important trait I bring to how I work with clients. Which qualities are most important in to you in your situation? Complete the worksheet in the appendix after you read the list below.

Qualities of Being a Practitioner That I Value

—I'm excellent at listening with my whole energy field, noticing what arises in me, and what "jumps out" at me in the client's energy field. In session, when and if it's appropriate, I may ask clients to go to that area in their own body with their awareness, and see what we discover, what consciousness is held there. (I'll teach you how to do this in Part III of this TTC Method.)

—I'm skilled at "translating"—that is, describing precisely what I'm doing with clients in a way they can understand and take to the other members of their healthcare team (such as their physician, psychiatrist, or psychologist), to improve their care.

—I'm good at "translating" in another way, too, and that is, different terminologies. I can translate terms, etiology, effects and side effects, indications and contraindications—between conventional, allopathic medicine and the world of healing. These two worlds may describe the same phenomenon very differently; each modality brings something useful to the puzzle. When coordinated, insight into etiology and treatment and care all improve.

—Different cultures have different conceptions of health and illness, successful treatment, and sometimes even cure. I'm good at "translating" these different ideas of health and illness across cultures. People in traditional conceptual frameworks of medicine in Latin America, for example, have different ideas about medicine and illness than people do in the US. Ideas of what constitutes health in India differ from the same in the EU. These are just some examples of cultural differences.

—As in this book, I can describe and teach what energy is in a way that makes it palpable for people.

—I like to ask open-ended questions that help people "connect the dots" and understand organically what happened before that may have contributed to the health or emotional issue they now face. I don't believe in imposing what I sense on anyone; instead, I ask these open-ended questions so clients can discover for themselves what is true for them.

—I bring my full presence to client sessions. I'm human, obviously, and I commit to being as focused as possible with the fellow human being before me. I remember the details of what clients share with me, and I take notes. Over time, this helps with what I described above—the person can start to see the pattern of what they're working with, along with what's shifting in their lives.

—Process can be held "lightly," as though it's a fundamentally joyful activity to come to know oneself deeply. By this I mean I help facilitate the deep emotional work that is the reason a client has hired me, but I don't feel there's anything wrong with them or that there's anywhere else to "get to." This is news for some people, especially when they're in a lot of emotional pain, and may feel somehow "broken," or as though they, as one client voiced, "should be able to cope. Others do."

By holding a person's process lightly, then the work becomes a practice of self-discovery and just one aspect of life. In other words, someone can cry deeply with me, and then, for example, right after the session, go out to dinner with friends, and have a lovely evening. People don't have to get mired in personal process even as they go deep in understanding themselves.

—Because of the sensitivity I've been describing, I'm able to sense the energy in a room, both of individuals and a group; I can name this and describe it when it's relevant in people's interactions, for example in working with couples or in corporate meetings when such awareness is useful and why they've hired me. I also use this ability to connect with my audience when teaching and speaking.

These are the qualities I bring as a practitioner.

If you're the practitioner, what qualities do you bring? If you're the patient, what qualities do you look for in your practitioner?

Now let's look at the qualities in being a patient, or, if you're the healthcare practitioner, which qualities do you most enjoy working with in patients?

Qualities of Being a Patient That I Bring:

—Tenacity. I do everything I can to keep myself healthy and able to be strong enough to withstand any potential treatment, so I can live as well as possible, as long as possible. (This is a little like training for an athletic event when you're not an athlete. It means having a positive intention to choose to take actions for your long-term well-being as much as possible. We'll explore what I mean by this in great detail in the chapters that follow. It does not mean to be harsh with yourself or expect yourself to do things you could always do in the past, which you may not be able to do now. Instead, it means tracking inside yourself, moment by moment, where you are, and what you need, and then taking actions for your well-being based on what state you actually are in, right then.)

—Proactive intelligence. If something bothers me or I'm worried, I treat that as valuable feedback. I try to get underneath the initial panicky feeling to the root of the worry, which reveals the underlying need, and then I treat that need as a problem to solve. If I can meet that need somehow, I feel better and stop obsessing. I believe considering my worries as a puzzle of needs to solve has kept me alive longer than if I were not proactive. It's an act of self-love (in the positive sense) to treat your feelings as a sign you need something, or several "things," and then meet that need or communicate with people who can help you get your need met.

—Curious. I'm curious about the people who comprise my health care team. By that I mean I want to know my doctors, nurses, radiation technicians, my entire team as much as they'll let me, whether it's as simple as knowing what they did this past weekend, or knowing their hobbies, their beliefs, how they are on any given day. By nature, I'm a curious person, but it's also strategic: I want my care to be a partnership, and knowing my practitioners as fellow human beings both fulfills my curiosity about them as fellow humans and also allows me to trick myself into not obsessing about my own treatment, especially when I'm scared. See worry, above, under Proactive intelligence.

—Ability to witness. This one isn't always possible. But here's what it looks like when it is: I've learned how to observe my consciousness in various states and, as often as I can, to choose what to focus on, so I can choose what experience to have, what mood I want to be in. This helps me choose what I want to spend my energy on. (I'll teach you how to do this for yourself, too.) I can't always manage this, especially when I'm in a crisis of fear, or need to make a decision that will affect my life in an ongoing way, but this is a skill that can be learned. And just as with any skill, you get better at it the more you practice. Having some choice about the kind of experience I want to have even when I feel awful, helps. Sometimes that means I need to communicate my needs more clearly. Other times it means I need to binge watch TV. Other times it means I have to just surrender and go to sleep. Then James reminds me tomorrow is another day.

—Communicative. I'll share with my oncologist, radiation doctor, nurses, James, our families, and friends, what I notice, any specific needs I have that I can't fulfill on my own. This allows for the partnership in care that I just described above. Yes, I may be going through cancer treatment, but I want my dignity, too. Part of how I maintain dignity is to make the experience as pleasurable as possible. That means communicating, not stewing alone.

Using this list as a springboard, when you're the patient, which qualities are important to you, in both your healthcare practitioners and in yourself? When you're the practitioner, which qualities do you feel help you provide the best care possible to your patients? Knowing these qualities, you can communicate these to your patients. And what qualities do you bring? Turn to the worksheet in the appendix now called "Qualities Important to You in a Practitioner and/or Patient" and fill it out.

CHAPTER FIVE
WHAT IS ENERGY HEALING? AND THE NEW WAY OF WORKING AS A HEALER

I am rooted, but I flow.

- Virginia Woolf

What is Energy Healing?

Thus far, I've been using the term energy, and I referenced Barbara Brennan's description of energy like water in a creek bed. But I haven't yet defined "energy healing." The premise of energy healing is that everything you've ever been through in life is held as "cellular experience," or "cellular memory." Our cellular experiences are said to make a template, much like a blueprint. The premise of healing is that as you affect the template, that affects the way your energy flows, as well as your life experiences; shifting the template also affects the body.

You might think of this template just like a blueprint for a house. You cannot build a house without a blueprint; it's like a map which specifies exactly which materials to use where, the dimensions of each room, and every aspect of the building, from the foundation to the walls and roof, from plumbing, to electrical, to the surfaces of the walls, floors, ceilings and any built-in furnishings. It's the same with your body. If you change the blueprint, that changes the way the energy flows, which affects your life and your health on every level.

The template mirrors how we "run our energy" as we grow and mature, from fetal development in utero through birth, childhood, adolescence, and on into adulthood, as well as the dying process. By this I mean: Our life experiences affect how we allow our energy to flow or get blocked, how it becomes vital, strong in an over-compensating, defensive way, or weak.

To say we "run our energy based on our life experiences" implies this is also a model of psychophysical development. And so it has been considered in a long lineage of body-oriented psychotherapy—starting with Carl Jung, to Alexander Lowen, to John Pierrakos, to Barbara Brennan, and to those of us who studied with her and now are developing the branches of this tree.[11]

If this sense of running our energy and growing our physical bodies according to our experiences in life seems too abstract, think of someone you know who is thin, long-limbed, with bony legs, thin arms and long fingers, with a long, thin face and high arches in her feet. Can you picture this person in your mind's eye? Now think of someone you know who is less skinny, and whose weight is more proportional to her frame, and who has big eyes, keeps her head jutted forward, tends to roll her shoulders forward and collapses her chest. These two body types are likely easily recognizable for you; they can be true of males as well as females. You likely know someone who has the first body type and someone else who has the second type. Now consider someone you know who tends to be overweight, about whom people say, "He's a teddy-bear," big-hearted, and big all over. Now picture someone you know who is perhaps broad shouldered, with a strong upper body, strong chest and perhaps thin, stick like, less developed legs. This is the stereotypical body-builder's physique. Now envision someone you know who is well proportioned, where every aspect of his or her body looks harmonious, and who spends a lot of energy, time, and perhaps money maintaining his or her perfect appearance. These types are also likely instantly recognizable to you. Again, each type can be true of men or women. The theory is we grow into different, recognizable physical body types as a result of different experiences we have while growing up which affect how we run our energy. How we run our energy affects the template or blueprint that in turn shapes our body, both as we grow from childhood to adulthood but also throughout our lives. There are five of these body types, each with corresponding emotional issues that develop as a result of experiences that happened often as each person was growing up. The somato-emotional types are called "characterologies," and were originally named by Alexander Lowen and expanded on by Stephen Johnson, Barbara Brennan and others.[12]

While it is beyond the scope of this book to explore the characterologies in detail, that work is fascinating; the contributions of each generation's teachers in that lineage explore physical, emotional, mental, and spiritual integration in human development and evolution in ways I believe will be less marginalized and more recognized in coming years.

The New Way of Working as a Healer

When I first began my private practice and was in the "rose-colored glasses" phase of being a healer, I believed in healing as something close to a panacea. I was so excited by the possibilities of energy healing, and I witnessed such tremendous growth and results in my own life, and, after my training, then in my clients' lives, that I felt energy healing was something that could treat many ailments, as well as help with many emotional issues.

All of that assurance came crashing down when I got sick.

Crisis of Faith in My Modality

When I was diagnosed with cancer, as you can imagine, it led to a reevaluation of how I had considered energy healing. I moved from being a confident, idealistic healer to not trusting healing at all. I felt it could be useful for some minor conditions, like a sprained ankle, say. But mostly I suddenly came to feel it was all fantasy. I mistrusted my modality. I began to believe I could not in good faith talk about any aspects of healing with such enthusiasm, even as I knew and had seen the positive results.

Despite the fact that my doctors said I healed better and faster from my surgeries. Despite doing well on chemo overall. Despite being able to continue to exercise and ride my bike nearly every day except treatment days and the sick day a couple of days after each round. Despite anemia, I did comparatively well during treatment.

I no longer knew how to talk about any aspects of energy healing or the benefits it can and does confer. I didn't want to misrepresent healing or my own abilities.

The statements I had made so glibly in the past to clients who wanted to feel better, like, "healing could work with chemotherapy to keep chemo in the body specifically where it was needed and remove it from where it would harm the healthy cells,"—this now seemed preposterous to me.

Even the statements I had learned in my training that were not directly about healing, but represented similar values, then bothered me. (For example the position that "lifestyle modification could work," as I had believed so vehemently, now seemed ludicrous, as trying such shifts such as eating only raw food, wheatgrass juicing, cutting sugar out of my diet as much as possible, taking supplements prescribed by my functional medicine doctor—none of these had had any effect whatsoever on my rising tumor marker.) I had heard about other people getting good results with these, but they didn't work for me. I was in a real crisis of faith, though "faith" is not quite the right word, as Brennan had never asked us to take anything blindly, but always to look for confirmation from several ways of perceiving and most important, from the client herself. Yet I was absolutely lost, with nothing that I had believed in fitting anymore. I felt like I no longer knew who I was.

In the chapter on discernment I'll share more details about what I tried and how I learned the hard way to assess what was efficacious and what not.

The years of questioning helped me refine this Thriving Through Cancer Method, and not only for clients undergoing life-threatening illnesses. Now I mostly work with clients using the skills of this method, more than just giving healings. It's a partnership between the client and me as her or his healer. It's not usually hands-on, but involves more self-tracking on the part of the client, which I guide her in (and which I'll share with you, so you can do it, too). I find that this way of working doesn't involve the client being passive and me swooping down like some expert to do what I do to her. Instead, I work along with the client in helping her determine for herself energetic consciousness held in the area of presenting complaint. Let's unpack that healer-speak, and describe more precisely what I mean, so when I share with you how you can do this, too, you'll have a basis of understanding right from the start.

In the last chapter, we looked at what energy is and the premise of energy healing (that health is the free flow of energy and disease is blockage or depletion of energy). We discussed the energetic template that molds our cellular experience. Now on a cellular level, let's look at this more closely. What is "energetic consciousness"?

Have you ever observed a dog frightened by a thunderstorm? The dog typically shakes and sometimes howls any time there is thunder. Sometimes he'll hide under the bed, or in a closet, or in some dark, solitary place. This is energetic consciousness expressed as fear. I imagine if we could measure, during the storm, the dog's heart rate, respiratory rate, perhaps levels of inflammation, we would find the dog is having a flight reaction. Some clever person has invented a device for dogs who suffer from this fear during storms or fireworks, or who have anxiety when their human is away. It's called a "ThunderShirt." Essentially, it's a piece of fabric that fastens securely around the dog's body and "hugs" him tightly. This has been shown to help the dog stay calm.

In people, an example of energetic consciousness becomes clear when we discuss blindness: Have you ever accompanied someone who has recently become blind as he walks? His whole body is braced with every step. The muscle tension and tension on his skin is palpably clearly greater than in your own body. This is cellular consciousness, too, and if we measured in that moment, it's likely we'd see markers of anxiety such as heart palpitations, shallow breathing, sweating, and perhaps trembling.

As a practitioner, I work with clients to help them learn to track such areas of cellular consciousness, and to explore what's held there, like memories, dreams, and past experiences, just to name a few possibilities. As we explore and learn to stay present with whatever we discover, with no demand that what we uncover be different than it is in that moment, it begins to organically shift. The client learns a whole set of useful skills that she can apply to her whole life. This returns the client's power back to her. I'm no longer the expert, and she is no longer passive, wanting me to "fix" her with my perceptions which she might feel must be more accurate than her own.

Instead, we're allies; I guide her into discovering her own experience, and then I teach her ways she can choose to work with it. I'm there as her guide and mirror, and I resonate to allow her to feel what she's feeling (more on that in the next part). I love working this way, and clients report similar results to my former way of working—they feel better, their lives improve, they start to live more aligned with who they are.

So far, we've explored the need for the Thriving Through Cancer Method using my own life as an example—a jumping off point so you can perhaps see your own story reflected here, and can consider your own life and the factors that may have kept you split from the true unity of your mind and body perceptions. This rift is why there is a need for the Method on a personal level.

Now let's look at the need to heal the mind-body split from a larger, societal perspective, and talk about how, in order to grow in our abilities to perceive, and so to live our lives congruently with all our abilities integrated and available to us, we may need to disconnect to connect.

CHAPTER SIX
THE NEED FOR THE THRIVING THROUGH CANCER METHOD FROM A GLOBAL PERSPECTIVE

My heart is so small
it's almost invisible.
How can You place
such big sorrows in it?
"Look," He answered,
"your eyes are even smaller,
yet they behold the world.

- Jalaluddin Rumi

All know that the drop merges into the ocean,
but few know that the ocean merges into the drop.

- Kabir

The Need for the Thriving Through Cancer Method

While I've shared a lot of my personal story, around cancer, yes, but also around growing up in my intellectual family, I know from working with clients and teaching, that I am far from alone in this experience of disconnecting from my body's way of knowing.

So as we move into considering this schism from a more societal perspective, let's start with you—right here and now.

Do you know that feeling when you're in some beautiful, relaxing place, such as on vacation, for example, and you feel, "This is so peaceful and soothing!" And you try to enjoy it, yet somehow underneath, you feel restless, like you should be "doing something"? Or do you ever feel, when you get to relax, underneath the demand to do something, a feeling of exhaustion? Like it was so much effort to get to this place where you can relax, that now that you've arrived, you just feel very tired, like it's an effort to do anything? Isn't this the truth of how our lives often are now: We finally have some downtime, and we find we're so drained, it takes a while to actually get back in touch with our own rhythm and recharge?

So, let's look at this question from the perspective of comparing: What is your daily life like? How much of your life is just like being on vacation? Probably not a lot, right? Instead, is your daily life busy or hectic? And do you love your life, but find that you sometimes feel overwhelmed, or tired, or agitated, cranky, scattered, like you just don't have the bandwidth to keep up with everything coming at you?

Let's take this a little deeper now. In the earlier chapters, I described my sensitivity. As you read, did you identify with my experiences? Are you also sensitive? Are you, too, an empath? Do you feel like being that sensitive is a lot to handle? If this doesn't seem like you at all, hold on; I think I may have an understanding of your experience, too.

Do you follow the news or politics in the world? Or do you choose not to, and it's a conscious choice not to, because—name your reason—but essentially, it's too much to bear, and you don't want to be so affected, or "give in to the negativity," or "bring your energy down"?

Or, here's another way of saying it: Numbness. Instead of feeling hypersensitive, do you often feel numb? As though you're the opposite of sensitive, like you don't feel much of anything? For example, does the internal monologue in your consciousness run something like this? "It's hard enough to work all day, and take care of the kids, and the spouse or partner, and it's really hard to get everything done, and by the end of the day, I'm just wiped out. I don't have time or the bandwidth to be affected by the news or by "stuff" happening somewhere else, to other people." Sound familiar?

And then, do you find that if and when you do happen to connect, it affects you deeply, and it's just too much to hold; you find it overwhelming. Can you relate to that?

Here's one more possibility: Do you meditate? And if so, when you do, how do you feel? I imagine it helps you feel unified, and you feel great. Or if you're a healer or healthcare professional, when you see your clients or patients do you feel exhilarated, connected, expanded? But then at other times, do you feel your life goes back to being busy, really busy, overwhelmingly busy, and you feel cut off from yourself and others, like you don't behave in ways you want to? Like you don't behave congruently with who you believe yourself to be?

Do you spend a lot of time online—texting? emailing? reading various websites or blogs? Do you play games? Surf online? Shop incessantly? Look up recipes? Watch movies endlessly? Do you ever "fall down the rabbit hole" such that Facebook becomes like what TV was a generation ago—hours can go by before you even notice?

Is this a familiar experience?

I think you get the idea with all my questions—when you relax, or do your best work, or connect spiritually, maybe you feel expanded, content, aligned with who you are. But for many, many people, this feeling is not at all what our daily lives are like. Our ordinary experience, and see if this resonates for you, might be more like this:

Picture your family on vacation. You're in some beautiful place. You've planned it; you've arranged the time when your whole family can go, you've gotten everyone packed and unpacked, settled in, you're there, ready to enjoy the beauty and... what happens? Everyone tends to gravitate to his or her respective electronic device.

I first became aware of this tendency when my family was in that situation. There we all were—the two of us, James' parents, his brother, his brother's wife and kids, and we were about to go for a beautiful hike, when James took a family picture. Everyone was sitting together in the living room of this elegant-rustic timeshare. We were clearly enjoying each other's company: Jackie, then age eleven, was sitting on the arm of the chair where Mike, her stepfather, sat. Jackie's brother Deon, their mom, Gina, and my "California Mom," Dee, all sat on the couch together. And every one of us was on an iPhone or iPad. Our heads were jutted forward, we were each engrossed in what we were learning.

So that's just it, right? We were in contact with each other a little bit, in that we enjoyed being in the room together, and we were connected to the larger world through whatever we were reading or looking at, each on his or her device of choice. Now, granted, this isn't what we do all the time when we're together, but—it happens. Often.

Does this sound familiar to you?

This is what life is like today. We have the potential to know, in nearly real time, what's happening all over the world. We see the pictures, and we feel a lot. We take that in. If we're empaths, we feel it in our own bodies.

I ask you all these questions because I feel we live in this age where the promise of technology is to connect us all, to potentially join all living beings on this planet, and surprisingly enough, we find it's having the opposite effect: we don't feel at one with everyone or sometimes, with anyone. All our hours on our devices tend not to help us feel more unified.

On the contrary, spending time this way seems to make us feel frustrated, tired, like there are all these other "things" we "should" be doing or attending to or doing differently. Or we feel angry and powerless to change the suffering we see and feel.

As I write this book, I notice this tendency in me. I keep wanting to check email or distract myself by looking at fashion blogs or Facebook. This is just how it is lately. But I meditate! And pride myself on being someone who can focus easily. But maybe that was more true of a past version of me than my present self.

So, what about for you? If you're feeling overwhelmed, agitated, scattered, forgetful, irritated, angry, tired, wired, pulled in a million directions, first I want to let you know, you are not the problem. It's not your fault. It's not like if you could just be less sensitive you'd be able to handle this onslaught, the bombardment. No.

The fact is, we're caught in a change. Life is like this now. It wasn't like this, to this degree, even ten years ago, in 2006. I know, for example, when I used to teach at the Barbara Brennan School of Healing, the amount of emails I started getting from students by 2010 made my job much more time-consuming than it had been just a few years earlier. This technology—emailing, the Internet—wasn't even available for most of us twenty years ago.

And the reality is, we can't go back. We can't revert to that simpler time of fifteen to twenty years ago when we actually saw our friends in person and didn't mostly "see" them on Facebook; when, if we were in the same room with family, we would all do something together. And I don't mean to yearn for some imagined "good old days." I'm shocked to remember as I look up when this all began that the change has actually been so recent. The promise of the technology has—this fast—become part of our lives; and we're not Luddites—we can't imagine our lives without it.

So if you're feeling overwhelmed, I'll say it again, in case you were too scattered in reading (as I often am lately) to let it land the first time: You are clearly not alone. And it's not your fault.

So, that's the problem: We're all disconnected from ourselves and "differently connected" with each other. And even if we know how to quiet our chattering minds, and align, such as when we meditate, or when we work with clients or patients, or when we're feeling well and not worried, if we're the patient, but then life takes over and gets hectic again. And so there's this dance that happens: Sometimes we're congruent with our sense of being our best selves, demonstrating our full potential, and other times we feel frustrated. And underneath it all, I think there's a feeling of "Mercy!" We know somewhere inside we're never going to be able to keep up. And yet we still long for contact, both with ourselves and each other.

So, what if in the middle of all this, you had a way to connect with yourself? And I don't mean those times when you meditate or you're trying to be mindful. Those are great.

But this is the dance between who we are when we're our optimal selves, and who we are when we're overwhelmed, in defense, not at our best.

Our healthcare system reveals this dynamic often. It's continually apparent (especially in the US healthcare system), how challenging it is for doctors and nurses to have any shred of a possibility for self-care. The values that inspire and attract many to the field of medicine get ground out of countless excellent clinicians by the ways we've collectively now structured these professions. Already intrinsically demanding, medicine as it's practiced now in the US is a system that I doubt can be maintained for practitioners for more than a generation.

And patients face the same problems in their lives, though differently. But when they're sick, and newly diagnosed, and scared or angry, this issue of disconnection from oneself and each other reaches a fever pitch. That's part of why there's such a split between conventional allopathic medicine and alternative treatments: patients want to believe they can feel better easily. Underneath is a fear that we can't control our own life, health, and death. Which is ultimately true, of course for everyone. But that's a difficult awareness to maintain when you've just been told you might not live so long.

So what's another possibility? Let's discuss it first in more general terms and then we'll become more and more specific. Let's take chemo nurses as an example. If you're that nurse, what do you do when you're at work, and the alarm on a patient's chemo pump button starts to beep, and meanwhile the doctor calls you to release the test for the blood you just drew, and the phone at the nursing station is ringing. And in the back of your mind you're thinking, "I hope my kids cleaned up their football cleats from the front hallway!" And "Boy! I'm hungry again. When's lunch?" Immediately followed by "Okay, remember not to eat too much..." Does this endless chatter sound familiar?

So, what if there was a way, if you're that nurse, that you could connect with yourself, on your feet, in the middle of your busy life? What if there was a way to know, moment by moment, how you actually feel, on every level—physically, emotionally, mentally and spiritually?

And what if you could learn how to be that in touch with yourself quickly and easily?

So you had the means to track inside your own body and energy field what you feel, such that you could be filled with that knowledge, and make decisions based on what you sense. If appropriate, you could communicate your needs to other colleagues directly, because you trust what you perceive, and know that there's space, within the culture of where you work, that sharing your real needs would actually be welcome.

This I believe is the antidote to what ails us: We need to learn how to be deeply connected to ourselves, and each other, through tracking our energy. When we can do that, we can be fully present, no matter what's coming at us. The alarm on the chemo drip can beep, the doctor can walk by and need something right at that moment, we can think about lunch, and it's all fine, part of the delicious flow of life. In fact, it can all feel gratifying, enriching, enlivening. What I call the "joy of presence"—that can be our life experience. As you learn this, and we'll learn how to sense this way in the next chapter, that skill alone has the potential to profoundly transform your sense of yourself in your life.

So now let's take this to a deeper level. What if that method for connecting with yourself and tracking inside also fosters your connecting with others?

I mean, let's say you've mastered how to do this, and you're in the flow—you're able to hold everything, be present without getting overwhelmed. As you go through your daily life this way, you can feel like some kind of superwoman or superman—joyfully present, and people around you will likely start to notice a difference in you. They'll recognize you're content, genuine, authentic, joyful, able to hold a lot, and not get burned out.

Now let's take this consideration deeper still. What if you know how to share this self-tracking and way to communicate your needs? That is, what if you can teach others how to track themselves, for example, people you care about: Your partner? Your colleagues? This can be a tool to allow the team to respect each person's unique contributions, value people, and so respect their needs. It can make the team coherent.

And now, envision for a moment: What if you can share this method with your patients? Picture how this can transform healthcare—if you're the nurse, or any healthcare practitioner, imagine what effect this can have on both your life and your patients'. Let's say there's a patient with a life-threatening illness, and she's overwhelmed by her diagnosis, and by how she's feeling physically. She has a lot of questions, and a lot of feelings. She may be terrified, or angry, sad, or all of these. What if you can share with her this way to track how she's actually feeling, moment by moment, so she can communicate to you directly what she needs? And she can hear the protocols for treatment, and choose what she genuinely wants, taking into account what might be actually efficacious.

Can you imagine, can you envision, what your work—your work to help patients heal—can be like then?

So far, we've painted this picture for a nurse or another healthcare professional. But what does the situation look like if you're the patient? If you're the one facing cancer or any life-threatening disease, imagine if there was room for you to bring this fully-present self to your appointments with your doctors and nurses. You can come with all your questions, your ideas, the alternatives you are considering or already using. You'd feel free to share your beliefs and values, your feelings about your diagnosis, as well as all your symptoms, emotions and concerns. Imagine there was time in the appointment and space for all these aspects whirling around in your conscious awareness.

If you're someone who has already figured this out, and you've found practitioners who can be present with you through the morass of uncertainties just mentioned, that is excellent. Yet in my experience both as a patient and a practitioner, and in anecdotes doctors tell, I hear many stories of how the doctor and patient do not always automatically see eye to eye; therefore the patient stops sharing information and concerns with the doctor. This is particularly glaring with the use of supplements or alternative treatments that can and often do affect conventional chemo medications. But it's also true in assumptions practitioners make about patients' choices regarding surgery, sexuality, religious beliefs, the dying process, and other sometimes still surprisingly taboo subjects, given the diagnoses. Even if a doctor believes he or she is knowledgeable about how to be sensitive to different values, the year-in, year-out number of patients who are unwilling to consider what you as a physician know can help them, can make these conversations trying. And unlike therapists and some modalities of healers, doctors and nurses are not required to be in ongoing professional supervision, so they do not have regular support around how to have these conversations.

So, again, if you're the patient, what if you can teach this way of sensing to your healthcare team? So that their jobs, their ability to serve you and help you stay alive, also becomes an opportunity for their growth? Then your interactions and conversations become both a reflection of and a way to practice self-care—in other words, you truly become partners. Can you imagine what your doctor's appointments can be like then?

Let's describe this more concretely now for both the professional and the patient. What if you can learn to use your own body, your own energy field, as a listening device? If you're a healer or aware of the impact of your touch, you may likely already have the common experience that when you put your hands on someone, you get so much information. What if every moment of your life can be like that?—without you needing to put your hands on anyone. And not in a way that's overwhelming, where you're taking on your client's "stuff," but instead, you're resonating, vibrating, fully present, and at the same time, you've taught the patient or client how to do that, too. Then there's nothing to fix, no need to save them, no need to do anything massive, or anything at all, really. Instead, you can just be, together. The protocol is likely to be the same; the tasks and actions may be identical. But the quality of your interactions, the richness of your conversations, the nuances of putting forth a treatment plan while you check for the patient's responsiveness or not—these are deepened.

And if you're the patient, as you hear these recommendations, and as you research, you can sense your needs inside. And rest yourself into the accuracy of what you perceive, and communicate those needs to the trusted members of your team. Can you feel what that can be like? Can you sense how that might have the power to transform your care and healthcare in general? Where you are truly empowered, and your care is a partnership, it's a win-win situation. It touches on the simultaneously wonderful sacredness and ordinariness of our human ability to connect with one another.

With these skills you can also feel less afraid and less victimized by your health challenge, but instead choose to work with cancer or any life-threatening illness as a vehicle for self-growth, even as you go through often grueling treatments.

Now from the most minute level of detail: From this place, every interaction, every conversation, every blood draw, every dose of medication passed from nurse's hand to patient's in the little plastic cup, every noticing the crinkle in each other's eyes, each is sanctified and natural, thrilling, moving, and just part of ordinary, mundane human life, all rolled into one.

This is deep presence. This is the joy of deep presence. This is the antidote to all our feeling frustrated, or overwhelmed or agitated, controlling, disconnected, burned-out. It's the antidote to feeling numb—like we just can't handle this much coming at us all the time, like we don't have the bandwidth.

Here—the supply is unlimited. We're connected with ourselves, connected with each other. Feel in your body what that potential feels like, and we'll explore how to get there in the next chapter.

This feeling, this way of being, this way of connecting with yourself, tracking moment by moment how you're feeling—is my passion. And as you probably can tell by my story, I'm obsessed with it because obviously, I needed to learn it; it didn't come easily to me.

In the next chapter, we'll move into the two parts of the Thriving Through Cancer Method. First, we'll look at the assessments you can do with and for yourself and/or for another. Out of the assessments, you learn what you need, so there are practices detailed in the chapters that follow the assessment tools, so you can meet those needs.

These tools, along with the practices I choose for myself at any given time, have transformed my experience of going through cancer into a very different reality than it is for so many people. And whenever I go to doctor's appointments—my surgeons, my hematologist-oncologist, the nurses I see every month—everybody says, "Wow! You're doing so well! What are you doing?" When I say to my oncologist, "I think I'm living longer and feeling better than other people," she nods her head vigorously, and says, "Yes, absolutely."

As I look around the waiting rooms, I can see it's true. I see other patients. And of course we identify with each other. As we sit together and wait to be called in to see our doctors, there's a curiosity, and a tendency to start talking and bond with each other in the first five minutes of a conversation, because we're all hungry to survive. Yet often as I look around,

I see how I'm having a different experience than my compatriots. We're citizens of the same "country"—the country of cancer, but it's like we come from different "planets." The assessments you're about to learn I developed because I needed to know precisely what I experience. The practices you'll learn, and then choose for yourself, I put together because they help me. It can be so for you, too. Without further ado, let's now turn our attention to the assessment tools of the Thriving Through Cancer Method.

PART III

--

THE TOOLS AND PRACTICES OF THE THRIVING THROUGH CANCER METHOD

CHAPTER SEVEN
THE ASSESSMENT

There is a force within which gives you life—seek that.
In your body lies a precious jewel—seek that.
Oh wanderer, if you are in search of the greatest treasure,
don't look outside. Look within, and seek that.

- Rumi

The Assessment

Now we move into the essence of the method.

So far, we've framed the Thriving Through Cancer Method in a few ways: We started the book by considering this period in our understanding of cancer as being shaped by our new ideas about genes; I shared my personal story in the context of this revolution in the conception of genetics, which, not incidentally, parallels the popular use and sharing of information via the Internet. There are many ways that this genomic era can and will affect so many of us. Here are just a few examples: Whether one is confronted by the decision to test or not to test, or by living with the news of one's genetic status and elevated risk of certain diseases that accompanies positive test results, or, more concretely, with the knowledge of which genes are expressed in a tumor removed from one's body and then submitted for genomic analysis of that tissue sample—which then can and will be matched with current and yet-to-be developed drugs—these situations highlight the need for a method that can help one navigate through the emotional (and perhaps spiritual) terrain evoked by all that these new technologies promise and deliver.

We then moved into the story of my diagnosis with fallopian tube cancer fifteen years later, along with my treatments in all the gory details; but I've also voiced the fact that I've survived longer than statistics predicted, and am thriving despite multiple recurrences.

Next, we looked at the need for the TTC Method from both individual and societal perspectives: First, from a personal level, as a need to unify our minds and bodies—because many of us don't know how, or have forgotten how to draw on an embodied way of knowing, and we're certainly not in the habit of living that way. Then suddenly, when faced with a difficult situation like a life-threatening illness, we don't know where to begin to consider all the choices for our treatment and care.

From a societal point of view, we looked at the TTC Method as a skill that our current reliance on technology doesn't yet foster, even as we're evolving to be able to contain more and more knowledge and information, and potentially be more and more connected with our fellow human beings and all living creatures.

Now as we turn our attention to the actual method, we're going to start with the assessment, and then move into the practices.

This part of the book is the "heart" of the TTC Method, and as I mentioned, you can use it by yourself, with your clients or patients, and groups (such as support groups) can work the steps of the method together. You can also implement the method with your team, as we talked about in the last chapter, so the method can be used by nurses or physicians (or even, someday, by both together) in a group practice or in a hospital setting.

We've focused a great deal in this book so far on life and death issues, but developing the TTC Method so I could live as well as possible as I went through cancer is only part of the story. The truth is, since I discovered ballet at age ten, I had always dreamed that someday, when I grew up, I'd spend part of each day exercising in a way that helped me go inside and connect with myself; I'd spend another part of my day writing, and somehow I'd still have time to work, and see the husband I dreamt someday I'd be with (and am now, happily and much to my surprise, married to). Somehow, too, I'd also get to see friends regularly. I had wanted to live in this integrated way for what felt like my entire life. And, in case you hadn't noticed, I'm also someone who's drawn to notions of how to create an optimal life; I love the idea of being as fully developed a human creature as possible.

But before I got sick with cancer, I was shy about committing to live in this unspoken, but recognizably unified way. As it does in various ways for so many of us, cancer cut right through that reluctance. "No time like the present," grimly summed up my attitude as I began to commit time every day to checking in with myself, and then doing what my assessments told me would help me feel better.

But much to my surprise, I actually did feel better when I followed what I sensed I wanted to do. I mean that literally, not ironically. It's obvious, but honestly, I didn't know that I could spend my life-time, my life energy living the way I wanted to. I've heard from many clients going through cancer and other life-threatening illnesses that they can relate—they didn't know they had a right to spend their own life-time the ways they wanted to, either. This Method transforms that issue, by helping you get clear on how you want to spend your time and energy at any given moment.

I developed the TTC Method as a synthesis of every tool I know. It is an amalgamation of what I know as an energy healer, with what I learned in the years spent dancing, choreographing, acting, performing, writing, and directing theatre pieces. It includes methods from body-oriented psychotherapy, physical actor training from Jerzy Grotowski's "poor theatre," along with techniques I invented that worked for me through many situations—from the adolescent wish to lead a well-examined life, to coping with losing people when they died or we parted ways, to discovering my views politically, to learning what I treasure or can't abide in social interactions.

The TTC Method utilizes the most embodied, integrated ways to learn, and can be used by people who prefer various learning styles. The assessment tools and accompanying "toolkit" of practices work synergistically—meaning, you grow and evolve in each area of your life (physically, emotionally, mentally and spiritually), more than you would if you only worked on one area at a time. In other words, the whole is greater than the sum of its parts—all areas of your life develop. In practice, what this feels like is a sense of being engaged, then skilled, masterful, in fact, and you feel you have choice, which helps you feel you have dignity, no matter what you're going through. You can feel well-rounded, self-reliant, self-trusting, even as you accept treatment, care, and help.

The Method helps you live optimally because you tailor it to you. I encourage you to learn the tools of the TTC Method, and then adapt it— shape it in ways that support you. As I said in the Introduction, I'm not interested in having you just copy me; simply parroting goes against what this Method is about, which is coming to know yourself and your needs better.

The Assessment part of the Method in particular is a way to grow an interior sense of yourself and your lived experience. It's counterintuitive, but slowing down to notice your interior experience gives you the ability to handle more in life. You can contain more, respond more. (The result is everything we talked about in the last chapter: you know how you are, moment by moment, so you know what you need, and you can meet those needs, and can communicate your needs to others. If you're a patient, you can communicate with your doctor, nurse, loved ones, and friends. If you're the doctor or nurse, you can help your patients and your culture begin to foster actually communicating your real human needs, both from patients to you, and for you, among your coworkers and colleagues.)

If you work in healthcare, as we said, you likely already recognize that that is not how it is very often lately. Here we'll add that this is a new model of healthcare that fosters your own self-care as a necessary part of the equation in a specific way. From an energy healing perspective, your own listening to your needs *resonates* (and we'll discuss what that literally means as well as how to do that, below), it models to your patients that their own health, including healing and recovery, is possible. An environment that fosters your own self-care allows also you to be present for the uniqueness of each patient, rather than numb.

Two Aspects Comprise the Thriving Through Cancer Method:

1. The Assessment—a four-step tool you can use to know exactly how you are, and how your patients/clients are at any given moment along with their underlying needs; and

2. The Practices—physical, emotional, mental and spiritual. Based on what gets revealed by your assessment, you choose which practices meet your needs. You "do," that is, practice the practices. Then you reassess. Based on what your *new* Assessment reveals, you then choose the practices that fit your new needs. Thus, the Method becomes a feedback loop that helps you enjoy better and better quality of life.

In the course of writing this book, I interviewed oncologists, surgeons, and researchers. In my private practice, I've worked with many doctors, psychologists, therapists, nurses, massage therapists, and other healers. I also met several hundred nurses when I gave the keynote at an annual conference for nurses where I began to teach this method.[13]

One of the people I interviewed is John Barstis, MD, a hematologist-oncologist at UCLA.[14] He was my main doctor when we lived in Los Angeles. Dr. Barstis is brilliant, a creative, dynamic thinker, and an excellent strategist in the ways he approaches the personalized treatment of cancer. He's a deeply feeling man, and very funny, too. I believe he helped keep me alive by learning all the details of my case, and then suggesting (and offering me the choice), that we use Doxil for my first recurrence, thus jumping that drug ahead in the queue of which drugs to use when, in which order of recurrences. "Let's keep you strong, so you can take advantage of all the future drugs that are being developed," he said. As I learned that Doxil is relatively easy to tolerate, with less cumulative toxicity than other drugs, I fully agreed.

When I interviewed Dr. Barstis for this book, he said:

> "There's a lot we're learning, and a lot we don't yet know about what can aid cancer survival. If exercise through good cytokine release can enhance cancer-fighting survival, then so can other things." He went on: "Conceivably, the brain can do that, too. We're too crude in our understanding of the brain."

He continued,

> "It's fascinating to me as a person. I'm a sensitive person; I fight with my patients. I'm in the battle with them. How do you survive and try to thrive while you have cancer? Some people are going to live ten to twenty years with cancer. It's a drag. One of the ways, is to consider cancer like a nasty relative. It's like having a psychotic sibling that you're always having to be responsible for. That's true, but it's in the background, while you live your life."

This seems funny in a way that also makes me a little nervous. I can feel myself titter and fidget remembering the first time he said that, like, who can embrace that comparison, that almost inadmissible, hostile feeling of resentment at having to constantly deal with someone else's issues, which seem to have nothing to do with you, and yet which still impact your life fairly constantly? But the analogy feels exactly right, too. Cancer is always in the background, and sometimes it feels like, "Wait. How did I end up here? This isn't me; all these doctor's appointments have nothing to do with the real me." So yes, cancer is always in the background, but as often as possible, that's where it belongs. In between dealing with the "psychotic relative" of cancer, and for some of us, multiple recurrences, life goes on.

So now, as we move into the method itself, here are the five tools that comprise the Thriving Through Cancer Method. There are four steps to the Assessment. And then there are the Practices (physical, emotional, mental and spiritual). All the tools move from self to other, with a telescoping perspective from the narrow focus on the personal to the broader taking in of another or a group at the same time as oneself, to sensing and contemplating the cosmic and spiritual. In reality, this distinction is artificial, as the personal, narrow focus is the same as the vast perception of the cosmological. But living with such awareness as you go through your daily life, often takes practice and a reframing of your perspective.

The Five Tools of the Thriving Through Cancer Method Are:
1. Self-Tracking;
2. Self-Tracking and Tracking Other(s);
3. Assessment;
4. Resonance; and
5. The Practices.

Let's explore these in more detail. Each can be understood in a little more depth by the following:

1. Self-Tracking: is what we've been discussing so far throughout this book. It's a means of observing what's happening inside yourself physically, emotionally, mentally, and spiritually;

2. Self-Tracking and Tracking Other(s): As you sense yourself and the other (or others) at the same time, you learn to treat as everything as "in," that is, relevant to the present situation.

3. Assessment to Foster Discernment: By listening in the two ways above, you learn the state and worldview of another (or others);

4. Resonance: as a listening tool, including two "scores". By "score," I mean like a musical score used by an orchestra conductor. That sheet music has different lines for each instrument in the symphony orchestra. In resonance, the two scores of what to focus on are:

   A. Words and tone; and

   B. Body language and energy;

That is, you pay attention to the words being spoken, and also, at the same time, to the feeling underlying the words. Sometimes these will be congruent, and other times not. Both scores are relevant.

5. The Practices: These organically emerge from listening in these ways.

CHAPTER EIGHT
SELF-TRACKING AND TRACKING OTHERS

The only journey is the one within.

- Rainer Maria Rilke

Self-Tracking

Now let's move into the step by step experience of each of these tools of the TTC Method.

The first step is to take a baseline reading of where you are right now, before we begin to use any of the tools. You do this so you can notice what shifts as a result of working with any of the tools. This can be done sitting, standing or lying down. Just by paying attention to yourself right now, in this very moment, what do you notice: Are you sitting? Standing? Lying down? How's your breathing? Shallow or deep? Any areas where you have physical pain or tension? If so, where? What's it like? What mood are you in? How are you feeling emotionally? How's your mind? Any "chatter" going on? Anything you're obsessing about? Any awareness of how you're feeling spiritually at the moment? Connected and unified? Not unified? Anything else you notice?

There are no right or wrong answers here. You're just observing. This is your preliminary sense of how you feel right now, before you do anything else. As we start to work with the first tool, Self-Tracking, you may notice that you feel different after you do it.

If you wish, turn to the worksheet now in the Appendix, called "Your Baseline Before Self-Tracking," and fill in your answers to these questions. You can compare your "Before" answers (now) to your "After" answers once you've done the Self-Tracking.

Self-Tracking is the foundational skill of the TTC Method. First you're going to learn how to do it inside yourself. Then you're going to learn how to track inside yourself, and track someone else at the same time. Then you're going to take what your self-tracking reveals to you, and assess which areas of your life can benefit from some support and what kind of support. Then we'll explore how you can use resonance as a tool to listen, and also how to use it to help clients or people "drop into" their real feelings, especially if they're stuck. Then we'll move into how you can put your practices together into a "menu" or "toolkit," and then into the practices themselves.

Self-Tracking

This fundamental skill cuts through all the chatter, all the distractions and "noise" in life. No matter what you're doing, this is the tool you can quickly use on your feet, in the middle of anything else. It allows you to quickly make contact with yourself and know where and how you are, moment by moment.

It relies on a specific skill, the ability to use one part of yourself and your conscious awareness to notice what's happening in another part. That's what I mean by "tracking." It's like following something or someone based on clues—like following an animal in the woods from the footprints left as the animal walked a path. Body-oriented psychotherapist Susan Aposhyan calls this "intrasubjective intersubjectivity." She writes,

"In the psychoanalytic world there is interest in exploring the intersubjective space between two individuals. This refers to a shared, mutually created aspect of relationship and includes intimacy. I use the term "intrasubjective intersubjectivity" to acknowledge the internal relational space that we can create by attending with one part of ourselves to another part."[15]

The first few times you learn it, practice in a peaceful environment, so you can get good at using this tool. Once you've gotten used to it, you can track yourself standing up, sitting, or lying down, at any time, anywhere.

So now sit in a chair with your feet on the floor, your spine straight, away from the back of the chair. Again, once you've practiced this, you won't need to be so formal about it, but for now, learn it with this detailed level of focus.

You want to make sure your spine is straight. How can you tell if it is? Pick up a piece of hair from the top of your head and lift it straight up, until you feel a gentle tug. This will give you a sensation on your scalp. See if you can feel a connection between that spot, on the top of your head, all the way down to your tailbone at the base of your spine. If you are bald, gently tap on the top of your head, and see if you can feel the connection with your tailbone. Feel free to experiment with where the correct place is on your scalp to tug some hair or tap on your scalp so that you feel the through-line. If you can't feel the connection all the way down, see if moving your pelvis helps. You might rotate your hips, and tuck your pelvis under and then release it a few times; then tug on a piece of hair or tap on top of your head again. See if you can now feel the connection all the way from top to bottom and vice versa. If you can feel it a little bit, notice how far down you can sense the connection. Move that part of your body, and see if that helps you feel a little further down. Keep checking in and moving each part until you feel it all the way down to your tailbone. If you can't feel the connection yet, that's okay; it gets easier with practice.

Now, notice what you're doing with your head. Are you someone who tends to hide a bit? Are you shy? Do you not always know your self-worth? If so, do you tip your head down? Do you tuck your chin in so your gaze is at the floor straight down in front of you by your feet? Let your chin be level, soften your gaze, so your eyes are open softly, and look at a spot on the floor about three feet (about a meter) in front of you. Let your head and neck be loose. If you feel any tightness in your neck or shoulders, you can move them, but don't do anything to try and make the pain go away right now, just observe it.

Next, notice what your pelvis is doing. Is it tipped backwards or forwards? You want your pelvis aligned directly underneath your torso and abdomen, as if you're riding a horse. If you need to adjust, do. (And if in the future you do this standing up, make sure your knees are bent directly over your feet. You will likely want to turn out your toes slightly to make sure when you bend your knees they bend over your feet. This protects your knees from strain.)

We're going to approach Self-Tracking from a physical and emotional perspective. Here are the steps:

Physical

Envision a ball of light glowing above your head, above your crown chakra. (We'll define and discuss the chakras more in the practices section of the book.) If you'd like, you can jump ahead and learn about the chakras first and then come back here. If you want to practice this now, before you get to that section of the book, that's fine. Just picture the ball of light above your head.

1. Allow the ball of light to enter your body through the top of your head. If you know about the chakras already (and again, we'll explore them more in the practices), let the ball of light enter down through your crown chakra.

2. Endow that ball of light with senses: Allow it to see, feel, hear, taste and smell and also know. Let it have conscious awareness.

3. Gently let the ball of light travel down through your body, sensing as it moves. Let it gently travel down through your head, down through your throat, down through your shoulders, down through your arms, elbows, your forearms, wrists and hands, to your fingertips. Let it travel down into your chest, through your heart chakra between your breasts, down into your torso, your abdomen, your pelvis, your thighs, your knees, your calves and shins, your ankles, down into your feet and toes. (If you are a nurse or doctor, massage therapist, or a practitioner in any healing modality, and/or you know anatomy, you can explore through each of the systems of the body.)

4. As you allow the ball of light to gently travel down through your body, with its conscious awareness, what does it sense? Allow yourself to notice whatever you notice, with no demand for change.

5. You may notice a color, a sensation, a quality, an emotion. It may be literal, or it may be symbolic or associative. Whatever you notice is fine. Again, there's no right or wrong answer here, just observation.

6. This is especially important: If you notice an area of tension or pain, do not try to release it, or move, to make it not hurt. On the contrary, just notice whatever you notice. See if you can just be with what is.

7. Once you've scanned your whole body, go back to any area that draws you. Perhaps it's an area where you feel pain or tension. Perhaps it's an area that feels too open or "permeable." There's no right or wrong answer here. Feel free to go wherever you are drawn.

Somato-Emotional

8. As you go into whatever area draws your conscious awareness, continue to notice what you notice. What's there? What do you see? Feel? Hear? Smell? Taste? Just know?

9. Are there any memories there? Does a scene start to unfold in your conscious awareness? You might see it, hear it, smell, taste, etcetera. If so, what do you remember? Any associations? What does this remind you of?

10. Is there a way that what you're sensing connects with any issue you're going through or currently working with in your life? Particularly if you're going through a health issue, or an emotional issue, this may reveal itself to you. If so, what do you perceive? Again, this may be concrete, or it may be associative. Both are okay. Again, there is no right or wrong answer here. Just knowledge. Just insight.

A Few Points:

• You can do this alone, or you can do it with a partner, a healer, a nurse, doctor, therapist, friend, or fellow patient.

• Keep in mind you can ask questions of this area of your body. And then invite your body to "tell" you or "share with" you the answer.

If you sense answers, great. If not, ask questions of your body about why your body does not wish to communicate with you at this time. Notice whatever you notice.

Does your body need something from you before she or he feels safe enough and willing to dialogue with you? Start the conversation. Let your body know that even if you abandoned her or him in the past, you are here now and willing to listen. If your body wants something from you, see if you can give yourself that. If so, do so. If not, see if you can tell your body why not, and set a time when you can give your body what she or he is letting you know she or he wants.

Here's an example: Say your body says, "I don't want to talk to you because you never listen! You always work so hard and you never stop and rest!" Then you might ask your body, "Okay, what would feel better? I know I work too hard." Your body might say, "A nap!" Or, "Time to play!" or "I want to have dinner with a friend." If you can't give yourself what your body is letting you know she needs, see if you can tell your body why now is not the right time, but how you will give your body what she or he is saying she or he wants soon. And then schedule that in your calendar. So, in this example, you might say, "I can't stop and play right now, but I promise I'll take half of Saturday off this weekend. Would that feel like a good start? What would you like to do then?" You are building or re-creating an alliance between your body and the egoic, outer-directed self.

Now turn to the worksheet in the Appendix labelled *Self-Tracking: What Your Body Reveals* and answer the questions there about where in your body you were drawn, what you sensed there, using which senses? And if something was revealed to you that resonates with what you're going through now in life, make note of whatever you noticed. We'll draw on this material as you generate your practices.

Some Notes on Working with Trauma:

• What if, instead of your body not talking to you, instead, you get overwhelmed, and you start to re-experience traumatic events from your past? This happens sometimes in my practice, though it's uncommon. I want to give you tools here in case this happens. (Sometimes practitioners don't know how to handle when traumatic memories arise in clients. It's an important skill to know how to keep everyone emotionally and of course, physically, safe.)

If you're working this tool alone, and you start to panic or sink into a traumatic memory such that you are no longer aware of being in the present now, and safe, and fine, immediately stop what you're doing. If you've closed your eyes, open them and look around the room. Remind yourself you're in the present moment, and you're safe and fine right now. Stomp your feet on the floor so that you actually feel your feet, in the present moment, making contact with the floor. Feel your butt on the chair. Move your legs and buttocks if you're having trouble feeling the seat underneath you. Keep your eyes open and say things like, "I'm safe now. I'm here. I'm okay." You may wish to gently tap the palms of your hands against your thighs all the way down to your feet. Tap your feet, too. You're using your own hands to make contact with a part of your body that may not be aware you're okay now.

Experiencing strong feelings is not the same as re-experiencing trauma from your past. You may use the Self-Tracking tool and remember an experience that brings up a lot of feeling in you. For example, you may be drawn to a part of your body where you've had surgery. This may bring up intense feelings, such as sadness. You may burst into tears. That's just one example, and it's okay to cry. You are able to distinguish between the experience of surgery, and all that's held there and evoked by "going there" with your conscious awareness, from actually right now, being here, awake, and okay in the present moment. In healers' jargon, you're able to "hold both," and know that your body remembers that experience from the past while simultaneously knowing you're okay in the present moment.

Can you hear how that's different from how if you start to get lost in a traumatic memory, you lose the ability to know you're safe in the present? In the memory of trauma, you can't "hold both"—you sink into the memory such that it feels like it's happening right now, in the present moment. Needless to say, this is not beneficial, but re-traumatizing. That's why the steps I just described to bring you back to awareness that you're in the present moment now, and that memory is not happening to you now, are so important.

Once you're out of the overwhelming feelings, you can remind yourself and affirm for yourself, as Jung did, that we humans "have a gradient towards wholeness." This means we don't sense or remember what we're not able and ready to actually handle.

Then, the next time you do Self-Tracking, do it with a therapist or healer, or at least someone else in the room with you. That person should at the very least know that if you start getting nervous, or hyperventilating, or panicking, that they should take your hands in theirs and say, "Squeeze my hands. Look at me. Look into my eyes. Stay here. Right here in the present moment. You're okay. You're safe. We're here right now, and you're safe. Stomp your feet. Feel your butt in the chair. Right here, right now, you're fine. We're here together." This person should keep ensuring the client (in this case you), is making eye contact with them.

If you're the practitioner in this moment, you may wish to say, "I'm going to put my foot on your foot, so you know you're fine in your body, right here, right now, in the present moment.

(And then put your foot on top of the client's foot. It helps if you're not wearing shoes.) Or, similarly, "I'm going to put my hand on top of your head, so you know you are safe. Stay in your body. Stay here. Look at me; look into my eyes. Squeeze my hand." (Then put your hand on top of the client's head and bend down if needed, so you're at the same height as the client, and then look the client in the eyes.) These tools help the client stay grounded and "in" her body energetically, rather than ungrounded and trying to energetically leave, which sometimes happens if that's how she or he coped with disturbing or violent, dangerous situations in the past. Some examples of when this might come up include when someone has been sexually abused, assaulted or raped; when someone has been in a war; and/or is now a refugee; when someone has been in a natural disaster or witnessed terrorist attacks; when someone has been severely shamed or bullied. These are just a few examples.

• Self-Tracking is generally safe and an excellent way to deepen contact with yourself. It is contraindicated when a person cannot hold awareness of reality, and being fine in the present moment, even as one allows oneself to re-experience situations and events that caused pain in the past. Certain mental health conditions are also more likely to evoke such a response. These include psychosis, schizophrenia, bipolar disorder, severe depression. Please use your self-judgment (and professional judgment, if you're a practitioner), and do not do Self-Tracking if there is any risk of evoking feelings of trauma and you feel unprepared for how to be fully present as I just described and in other ways you may have learned from your modality.

This first tool, Self-Tracking, is powerful, and serves you as an individual. I'm a fellow traveler on this path. But each person has her or his uniqueness. The famous Martha Graham quote is relevant here (all but the narcissistic bit at the end):

> "There is a vitality, a life force, an energy, a quickening that is translated through you into action, and because there is only one of you in all of time, this expression is unique. And if you block it, it will never exist

through any other medium and it will be lost. The world will not have it. It is not your business to determine how good it is nor how valuable nor how it compares with other expressions. It is your business to keep it yours clearly and directly, to keep the channel open. You do not even have to believe in yourself or your work. You have to keep yourself open and aware to the urges that motivate you. Keep the channel open...No artist is pleased. [There is] no satisfaction whatever at any time. There is only a queer divine dissatisfaction, a blessed unrest that keeps us marching and makes us more alive than the others."

Remember how we defined health in energy healing as the flow of energy and disease as blockage or weakness or depletion? Self-Tracking is a way to perceive your places of vitality and flow in action, and observe your places of blockage, weakness, or stuck feelings. It's a powerful tool for self-knowledge, and even this act of observation alone, often begins to shift your interior sense of yourself.

If you want the truth,
I'll tell you the truth:
Listen to the secret sound,
the real sound,
which is inside you.

- Kabir

Self-Tracking and Tracking Other(s)

Now we're going to move onto the second Assessment tool: Self-Tracking and Tracking Other(s). As you grow comfortable tracking yourself, your capacity to observe both yourself and at the same time track someone else becomes possible. The "someone else" can be one person or a group. But for now we'll learn the skill for two people:

1. You—when you're the patient or client. I'll call this person the "client" now; and

2. The listener—(or healer, nurse, doctor, therapist). I'll call this person the "healer" now.

In real life, if you're currently a patient, you can work this tool from both perspectives: You can listen to your doctor or other healthcare provider as though she or he is the "client" and you're the healer. When you listen this way, you notice whatever you perceive about their energy, and you notice whether that's congruent with yours or not. This will help you assess your physician's recommendations for you. It can help you decide if this person is a good fit to be on your healing team.

You can also work this tool where you're the "client," and ask your doctor/nurse/therapist/other practitioner to be the "healer." Out of this, you may feel more in partnership with your practitioner, more integrated in your care, as you see that all your concerns can be discussed honestly.

In a support group, you can each take turns playing both roles.

One of the doctors I interviewed for this book is Arash Asher, MD. He is the director of Cancer Survivorship and Rehabilitation at the Samuel Oschin Comprehensive Cancer Institute at Cedars-Sinai in Los Angeles. In that role, he directs several programs. One helps prescribe rehabilitative physical exercise for cancer survivors after treatment is complete. That was how I first met him: I came as a patient concerned I might have neuropathy in my feet. (I fell several times in the months after finishing chemo the first time. My feet didn't feel numb, but it was as though my brain couldn't connect in real time to what my feet were doing. My legs were swollen with lymphedema, and despite tights, that made them heavy and big. As you can imagine, that upset me a lot.) With his kinesthetic way of sensing, I appreciated Dr. Asher's subtle mind-body way of checking what was happening with my limbs. (As I mentioned in the Prologue, I've since learned a tool to manage lymphedema so it doesn't bother me often anymore, and I'll share that with you in the physical practices below.)

Dr. Asher also co-founded a program to help patients with advanced disease address existential and spiritual challenges they may experience. Known as Growing Resiliency and Courage with Cancer, or GRACE, the five-week, structured, small-group program (there are seven to nine people in each series), encourages patients to discuss themes like wisdom, gratitude, courage, humor, and creation of one's legacy. The program includes readings, discussion, and learning a mindfulness practice.

These two different, yet related interests of Dr. Asher's reflect what we discussed—how doctors tend to gravitate towards specialties that mirror who they are as people. He described how it's the funniest "thing," but even as med. students, it's easy to know who will choose which specialty. Certain personality types are drawn to surgery, others to internal medicine. Rather than complaining that a particular doctor doesn't have a good bedside manner, he says, and I agree, patients can use the knowledge of what a doctor's personality is like as a way to check if that person seems like a good fit to be on your healthcare team.[16]

This second tool fosters that.

If you're the healer, it also allows you to help your client deepen into their real feelings, particularly if they're circling around, but not "dropping into" deeper material. With this tool, essentially, you're beginning to learn how to use your own body and energy field, along with that of your client, as an instrument, a listening device. Here's how it works:

Self-Tracking and Tracking Other(s) at the Same Time

1. The healer guides the client to scan through his or her body as described above in the first tool, Self-Tracking, above. That is, the healer says out loud the steps of letting the sensing ball of light travel down through the client's body. The client, meanwhile, follows those steps.
2. At the same time, the healer scans through the client's body and energy field, which both interpenetrates and surrounds the clients' body.

   1. What do you notice?
   2. When you get to the section of where you feel drawn in the body, both client and healer, notice where you're drawn.
   3. Client—let healer know where you're drawn. Healer—just listen. Don't share where you feel drawn yet.
   4. Healer, be curious: Does the area where *you* feel drawn correspond to the same area where the client feels drawn?
   5. If so, follow the client there, and step by step, ask client all the questions in that tool.
   6. If not, hold both simultaneously: follow the client there with your conscious awareness, and at the same time, remain curious about any area(s) that draw your attention.

7. Trust that what you notice is relevant, even if you are not working with that area directly.

8. Stay curious. As you ask questions with your client to help guide them into that part of the body/energy field, if/when it feels right, ask, "What about _____?" (the other part(s) you notice).

9. (This is the art of healing. Notice the timing. Do not ask when doing so will take the client out of process. Ask instead in a way and at a time that will further your client's insight.)

10. Very important! Be careful to not assume you know anything! In other words, don't "swoop down" like some "psychic expert," and act like you know what's going on and your client does not. Instead, allow the area that called you to be a jumping off point for further exploration and discussion. Always assume, as Jung did, as we mentioned in dealing with trauma, above, that there is a "gradient towards wholeness," that is, that your client's field will not reveal more than he or she can handle, and that your client knows him or herself better than you ever will.

11. At the same time you are holding the client, and what you notice in his or her field, now also at the same time, notice what's arising in you, in your field: For example: Are you hungry? Is your mind wandering? Are you distracted? If so, by what?

12. Instead of treating these as though you're somehow "bad" and lost contact with your client, instead treat these as further areas where you can be curious. Treat all of it as relevant. If you're hungry or sleepy or your mind is wandering, trust that that is somehow relevant to what your client is experiencing or unable to get to. For example, Is he having a hard time dropping into his feelings? Or, is she thinking she "should" feel differently, or is she judging herself? Is what she is saying triggering to you around something in your own life?

13. Trust that your client always, inevitably mirrors something in you, something you are also working on. In this, healing is a sacred art, a path for your own development along with that of your client. Healing grows the capacity for empathy, for feeling like we understand what it's like to be in another's shoes. You do not share that with your client, but you hold that awareness inside yourself.

14. If you're the client, you may wish to add any insight gained by working with your healer to the worksheet you started at the end of the last tool, the worksheet on Self-Tracking, in the Appendix. If you're the

healer, you may wish to make notes on a separate piece of paper or in a computer file about what you noticed in your work with this client.

So far we've mentioned how you can use this tool when you're the patient in checking out a doctor. And we've explored the tool where you're the healer and you're working with a client.

You can also use this as a way to listen at any time. You can use it in the classroom when you're teaching, in meetings, in any organization. This level of listening is profound because it is embodied. If you speak from the knowledge of what you're observing, it makes the connection between people deep—they feel heard and valued.

Chapter Nine
Assessment to Foster Discernment and Resonance

Very little is needed to make a happy life;
it is all within yourself, in your way of thinking.

- Marcus Aurelius

Assessment to Foster Discernment

This third aspect of the Assessment is a key tool and perhaps the most important step in the TTC Method, because it allows you to notice the worldview of another, and work with that person no matter if you naturally see eye to eye or not. If you're tempted to skip this step, don't!

If in real life you're a patient, this is the step that allows you to check if you're practicing discernment or falling prey to beliefs that may not serve you now. In other words, if you're the patient, you can use this tool to check in with yourself, observe yourself, and ask if you're asking the right questions. If you're the healer or healthcare practitioner, this tool allows you to serve your clients or patients, and check to see what they want from you, how they want to make use of your experience, skills, and resources.

As we move into this tool, I want to share a couple of stories with you. Before I do, I want you to once again take a baseline reading of where you are right now. That is, quickly scan through your body as we did before the first tool of Self-Tracking. This is your baseline. Notice now, in this moment:

How's your breathing? How does your body feel? What mood are you in? What emotions are you feeling? Note these on the worksheet on Assessment to Foster Discernment. (This worksheet starts with the same taking your baseline that we used before Self-Tracking, so you'll have space to write down your responses this time.)

You're taking your baseline now to see how you respond as you read these stories, so after you've filled out the worksheet with where you are right now, please come back here and notice these questions before you begin to read the stories. You'll be looking to observe: Do these stories evoke any feelings in you? How do you feel? Angry? Sad? Confident? Confirmed in your belief(s)? Doubtful? What happens to your breathing? Do you notice any shifts in your body, for example any areas of tension—does your stomach tighten, for example? Can you just observe any changes without any demand that you respond or not respond, or that you do it differently? After you've read the stories, please complete the second part of the worksheet on the Assessment to Foster Discernment. Here are the stories. Notice what happens in you as you read.

I bumped into a friend at a party. A woman about my age, she had recently been diagnosed with breast cancer. Known to be a teacher and a leader in her field, she was surrounded by people who were "yes-ing" her about her choices regarding her health. In her fear, with all her knowledge and wisdom, she was certain she knew more than the doctors she had chosen. But her breast cancer was a mass protruding from her chest, clearly growing quickly. As you can imagine, this visible lump was causing her a lot of fear and anxiety.

She had heard through the grapevine that I had been through cancer recently. She was eager to talk with me at the party, and her words poured out in a tumble. Everything in her training and belief system was convinced she could take certain steps, use alternative medicine, work through emotional resentments and disappointments, and make her cancer go away. People around her were offering explanations of what was happening in her astrological chart, things she was learning emotionally from this opportunity, etcetera. She was sure they were right. She was working with the belief they were right. After the party, she called me on the phone to talk. I found myself in the uncomfortable position of asking, "Have you asked if what you're doing is working?" Have you tested to see if your cancer is shrinking? Or is it growing?" She was angry. I felt terrible.

But a week later, she called to tell me she had changed her protocol. She had decided on surgery, chemo and radiation. She still believed everything else, too (what was happening for her astrologically, the emotional work she was doing to get over her disappointment and resentment about her divorce a year or so earlier). But she was now choosing the conventional medical path along with the other work she was doing. We wished each other well.

We didn't talk for a few years.

She emailed a few years later to say she was well. She had had one recurrence, but was again in remission and going on with her life. To me, her story is about waking up to using her skill of discernment. It was painful for her to suddenly feel she had to challenge her beliefs that way.

It was painful for me, too, both in the conversation with her, and in my own life, when I, too, had to surrender my beliefs, in order to make different treatment choices based on what was most efficacious. For me, too, coming to that awareness was a painful process—agonizing, surprising, humbling, undeniable. I'll share more of what that process was like for me in the chapter on discernment, below, but for now, in terms of learning how to work with this tool of fostering discernment, a few key questions are called for:

If you have cancer (or if a patient or client of yours has cancer), what kind of cancer is it? Is it aggressive or not? Does that type tend to respond well to chemotherapy or radiation or not? Do you have time to make up your mind which protocol suits you? Or must you decide in a hurry? Do you have time to explore alternatives if those draw you, even if they may work more slowly than conventional methods, or not? Usually when we're diagnosed, we go into panic mode. But answering these questions brings a clearer framework to your feelings, and potentially at least a little peace of mind.

But the stakes are high. Consider the other options:

I had another friend, with the same BRCA1 mutation that I have. When we met, we were both at a retreat center to learn about a specific alternative treatment. I was newly diagnosed, and had just had a hysterectomy, my first surgery. She was having a recurrence of breast cancer. She was a young-seeming forty-four year old—fit, radiantly beautiful, and otherwise healthy. She had three young kids, and was now in her second marriage, and very happy with her husband.

The alternative protocol we were doing made us both look glowing—our skin was shining, our hair looked great. (My hair hadn't yet fallen out, as it would do a few weeks later, a couple of weeks after starting chemo. Hers was growing back and was a short pixie haircut.) The regimen gave us lots of energy. I was there for a week. She had decided to do the whole three-week protocol.

The founder of this program gave lectures, and after one, during Q&A, I asked whether his regimen would work when someone has a genetic predisposition to cancer. He gave a lengthy answer that essentially included his belief system, which he put forth with great confidence: "If your tumor was 1.5 centimeters, you don't really have cancer. Your doctors are in the throes of Big Pharma." He guaranteed if I stuck with his regimen, I'd be well; my immune system would be strengthened and able to fight off the tumor-that-wasn't-cancer.

I remember after the lecture many people swarmed me. "Did you hear that?" an older man said. He had white hair, and a strong physique; he was a retired firefighter and still looked strong, even as he went through cancer. "You don't have cancer!"

It was so seductive, so tempting to believe the founder of that center.

I went home after that week determined to put into practice his protocol. I bought all the equipment to change my diet according to his recommendations. But I also did another CA-125 tumor marker blood test. And my number was creeping back up. It had been 164 before surgery, then dropped to 102 when I left for that week-long retreat after surgery. But it was back up—it was 170 after a week. Clearly, the cancer was not gone.

Much as I wanted to believe it was gone.

Much as I wanted to believe he was right, and I could simply stimulate my immune system and it would eradicate the cancer.

Much as I had heard testimonials from people for whom that protocol worked.

And having just had surgery, it alarmed me that the number was already increasing. I felt like I didn't have time to slowly deliberate, and see if the protocol would work.

Maybe it was the genetic predisposition; maybe it was the histology of the particular tumor that had been in my body, but it became clear that this particular diet and alternative treatment regimen was not working. I was forced to use discernment and change tactics. And it was not like I didn't keep trying. I did keep eating the way he suggested, and did follow the personal care treatments and supplements his team prescribed. But then my number kept increasing.

This was very hard! I'm a healer. It made sense to me with my training and values that if I bolstered my immune system, my body would eradicate the cancer.

But the blood test showed that diet wasn't having any effect.

My friend, meanwhile, had done the same CA-125 blood test before she came for the three weeks. Her results were already at 70, well out of normal range when she arrived (most versions of the CA-125 test in the US use either less than 21 or less than 35 as within normal range).

She did the three-week protocol, and (like me) believed in it. She looked so good! She felt great!

But she decided to "take the summer off, and not test until the kids go back to school in September."

In those three months, her CA-125 went from 70 in May 2012 to 967 in August 2012.

Why she chose to wait three months when she was out of range is mysterious to me. (Though I later did the same thing, when my doctor advised me that the trend in my marker was downward, and it was safe for me to go to Europe for three months; we'd repeat the test when I got back. For me, too, waiting that long when I was out of normal range had negative consequences. That led to the second, seemingly major recurrence, and, in a panic, when I got home and tested to find the number was higher than it had ever been before at 361, then two weeks later 660, I said yes to that huge surgery with the long incision, which, in the end, only revealed a small tumor.)

In any case, by the time my friend went back to repeat her tumor marker blood test three months later, she was having "little aches and pains" in her collarbone, and in her legs. Her CA-125 was then 967, the areas of pain were confirmed to be bone metastases, and at that point, it was too late. The cancer had spread so much that surgery was impossible and chemo could not keep up with it.

She died in February 2013, five months later, at age forty-five. She left behind her husband, two young daughters and a young son, her sister, her parents, and many friends. I still miss her, and I'm crying again as I write these words.

So you see, the stakes are high, really high—life or death.

It's tempting to believe what we want to believe. It's tempting to let our beliefs or values, our conditioning or our past experience guide us. It's easy to let how we're feeling physically be our only guide. But when there isn't much cancer in the body, it's possible to feel fine. As Dr. Barstis was fond of saying to me through my first two recurrences, "Melanie, you never had any symptoms from the cancer. Only from the treatments we've been giving you."

Yet just because I wasn't having noticeable symptoms, didn't mean the cancer was not growing. It absolutely was. That's why it's so important to get the diagnostics. This is not to say definitively that alternative methods may not be effective for some people and some tumors; I don't know. But I do know that it's of paramount importance to use the tools of diagnosis that conventional medicine offers. Then you can assess if what you've chosen is working. In the case of ovarian cancer, as we mentioned, it's called "The Silent Killer" because most women either don't have symptoms or the symptoms are so minor that we discount them.

It's so human to long to be well, and to believe what we want to believe will help us. If we know that our immune system defends our body against disease, it's extremely tempting to believe that if we simply bolster our immune system, it will be able to eradicate a cancer. (And with the new immunotherapy drugs being developed, that may yet prove to be true.)

It's so human to see something, want it, and draw conclusions. But when we're in the unknown, and our beliefs tell us one thing, and we're tempted to believe that's all we should base our decision on, this is when we can use this tool we're about to learn to call on discernment and ultimately ask, "Does it work?" If not, can we either make a new choice based on the information at hand, or be conscious of the fact that we're choosing this protocol anyway, and let that be our choice?

To be brutally blatant about it: The obvious question that we usually fail to ask is, can we let that be our choice, knowing we may die from our decision?

In the case of my friend in the second story, essentially, she waited too long. By the time she tested to evaluate whether her choice was efficacious, the cancer had metastasized to the point where conventional treatment could not work—certainly cure was not possible, but even a remission until some potential future recurrence (because of her genetic predisposition) also became out of the question because she waited.

Because she did not choose with discernment, she died quickly, and young. She is loved and missed. And this is happening and happening and happening, again and again and again. It seems everyone has lost someone to cancer. Many, many, many of us have gone through it ourselves. It is one of the signatures of our age.

We need integration between conventional allopathic medicine and alternative medicine, that is, we need complementary care when it works, and we especially need open dialogue and research. With the technologies available to us today, it should be simple—we need to share information— that's potentially easy, with the Internet—so people can make the best decisions, the decisions that meet their needs, that are not based merely on wishful thinking or beliefs and values irrelevant to the situation at hand. Initiatives in research are already being structured according to the new paradigm of researchers and labs sharing information. This is making research faster and obviously more collaborative. We need sharing of information clinically, too.

The tragedy of this disease is that it grows. It overwhelms the body. It's not that we humans don't have power, but that the rate of cancer growth ultimately outruns the body. We are not omnipotent. And sometimes cancer is more than we can handle.

So now let's turn our attention to the tool:

Assessment to Foster Discernment

1. Look at the first part of the worksheet you completed for this skill before you read the stories above, the baseline, on the worksheet Assessment to Foster Discernment.

2. Now fill in the second part of what you notice inside yourself as you read the stories above. What happens inside you as you read those stories? What do you notice? How do you feel? How's your breathing? Did any feelings come up in you—if so, which feelings? Complete the worksheet now based on your answers. Next we're going to take that knowledge and apply it to this tool.

3. For the next part, you can either use the worksheet you were just completing, and the one from the first tool in the method, the Self-Tracking worksheet, or, if you've been working with another person, you can use your notes from tracking with your client in the tool on Self-Tracking and Tracking with Other(s).

4. Look at whichever worksheets you choose now. Just like a doctor makes clinical notes, this time, we're going to be doing it after the fact, but as you get good at this, you can do it live and in the moment, either with yourself, or with your patients/clients.

5. As you look back on your notes from when you did the Self-Tracking and, if you did it, when you did the Self-Tracking and Tracking Other(s) at same time, now ask, about the client (who may be you):

6. What did you notice about the client's points of view or beliefs? Again, you can answer about yourself for all of these if you're the client. Or you can answer about your experience of your client.

7. Was she curious? Does she want to know more? Is she framing questions herself, or relying on you, the healer, to come up with or generate questions to ask her body?

8. Does she have good communication with her body, or was that difficult/challenging for her? For example, does she have trouble focusing on "listening" or "inviting" her body to share with the two of you?

9. Can she communicate with her body, but then not share that with you, so that she is silent for long stretches of time? Or is she good at communicating with her body, and comfortable sharing what she hears/feels/sees etcetera? Notice if she is attuned to her interior. Sometimes not speaking does not mean that she's not having a profound experience. She may be silently engrossed and not talking. Notice whatever you notice here. Ask her her experience.

10. Did she feel comfortable bringing back from the depths and sharing out loud with you what she sensed? If working the exercise alone, did you find it easy to write down/draw/give voice to what you sensed?

11. Can she stay focused (for example, by putting her hand on the part of the body she's focusing on), or does she keep "jumping out" of the exercise to talk about other things?

12. Notice what either state evokes in you.

13. Can you observe yourself observing the client, with no judgment?

14. Gingerly, keep inviting her back into deep contact with herself.

15. At the same time, ask, "How can I help you today? What are you looking for?"

16. Sometimes clients just want you to "fix" them; other times they're curious themselves.

17. How is that for you? Do you have any feelings she "should" be one way or the other? For example, do you think being "proactive" is "good"? and "just fix me" is "bad"? Or the opposite: do you feel it's more "work" for you to be present with someone who wants to know everything about what she's going through, when maybe you're in your own process, and would prefer to "not work so hard" or not have to be so present at this time?

18. What is the client mirroring in you? What might you be mirroring in your client?

19. Now here's a second part. If you're the client and you're working these exercises for yourself, answer the following questions about yourself now where you're the healer.

20. This time (turning the focus to you as practitioner), as you sense how the client did during the first Self-Tracking exercise (and if you did it, the Self-Tracking with Other(s) tracking tools), now notice what arises in you—

21. Just like when you read the stories above—How do you feel?

22. Do you want to fix the situation? Or give her resources? Or have her work with what got revealed for her in a specific/particular way?

23. Do you have a "charge" around this—meaning, you're sure your way is the right way? Meaning, do you have an opinion about which treatment she should choose?

24. See if together you can come up with ideas for how to meet her needs that were revealed by her self-tracking.

25. Without any charge or demand that she do things your way, offer the appropriate level of resources—you can know what that is by how she answers the question about how you can serve her today.

26. Does she want knowledge? Information? Strategies? Just deep contact? Support for a choice she's made out of her beliefs even if that doesn't utilize her discernment?

27. Match your tone and recommendations to what she tells you she wants.

28. If she is facing a life-threatening illness, see if you can both meet her where she is, and ask, gently, if she has a way to assess whether what she is choosing is working.

29. Gently draw a distinction between something seeming to work because we feel better and look better, and it actually being efficacious

which we can tell via diagnostic medical tests such as imaging and blood tests.

30. Express clearly that there are different ways of "working"—one method may "work" emotionally, but have no effect on the cancer (or other illness) (We'll explore this at length in the chapter on discernment, below.)

31. If there is no way to check if what she's choosing is efficacious, discuss whether she's comfortable with not knowing. Is she comfortable basing her decision purely on belief or what seems logical (e.g., if I boost my immune system with a particular diet, it will be able to eradicate the cancer naturally, without all the side effects of conventional treatment).

32. Ask if she'd like to know other possible options or ways of ascertaining if her choice is working. If so, assist in whatever way she asks to help her discover those. If not, respect that, honor that and do not foist other options on her.

33. If you see that her biases are getting in the way of her ability to have the conversation, affirm that she can make the right decision (notice if you want to say, "the decision that is right for her." Then see the next step).

34. Check if you have any demand or charge around wanting her to make a certain choice. If so, sometimes it helps to admit that that's your issue, not hers.

35. If appropriate, ask if it's all right with her for the two of you to have the "meta-conversation," that is, to share some ideas around the notion of discernment, and she can again choose to use these or not—take it or leave it—it's her choice.

36. Affirm again that she has the ability to discern what is right for her.

37. Ask if she is open to discussing the way that she can choose to use diagnosis to measure whether a particular regimen is efficacious. Again, you can support her in distinguishing between assessment of something being efficacious versus using some immeasurable (yet perhaps more important to her—and that's her right to choose) quality (for example, "I feel better now"), and basing decisions based solely on that.

38. Affirm that discernment coupled with her self-knowledge through this assessment, along with choosing the appropriate treatment for the situation at hand, helps create a coherency, a peaceful, empowered feeling. It cuts through fear. It allows one to relax into treatment. Even if it's hard to go through, there is a sense of "I made my decision based on

the best information I have, coupled with diagnostic testing. Everything is taken care of; I just have to show up and go through it."

39. Whereas before there is that clarity, there's often a thrashing around, trying to find what feels right, a desperation and willed hope. This is challenging.

40. Important! Again, notice what arises in you if her choice does not match what you would choose. Remember that your feelings about her choice are not your client's business. These are best worked with with your healer, in supervision.)

Forever is composed of nows.

- Emily Dickinson

Resonance

This is the fourth Assessment tool and the final one to use before the Practices. It can also be used in an ongoing way along with the practices. By definition, Resonance happens in relationship. You can't do it alone. You can practice with two people. Or you can practice in a group, such as a support group. But you cannot perform it solo.

(There is one exception to this, and that is if you imagine or envision yourself into a different state. Then you're working with different aspects of yourself, almost as if you're two people. Much like how an actor gets into character, as you get good at using Resonance, you can play with imagining one aspect of yourself—say a scared or worried part of you—is a different "character," who holds a certain vibration. You could try "acting as if," and play with changing your resonance or vibration as a way to change your focus and take yourself out of the state of worry.)

But for now, to learn the tool, we'll do it with two people. In Resonance, one person shares, and the other one listens. Obviously, as with all the skills, both roles can be either gender. In a group, you can adapt it so the listener is more than one person. For simplicity, we'll learn the skill with one person sharing and one person listening, and we'll describe here the one sharing as male and the one listening as female.

To summarize what we're about to do: The one sharing, who we'll call the client, can share about anything. He can share, for example, what he noticed during the Assessment to Foster Discernment. The listener resonates vibrationally, initially with what the one sharing is either experiencing or trying to get to.

What does this mean, to resonate vibrationally? As the person sharing begins to explore a particular situation, the listener pays attention to what is arising in her, just like in the second tool, Self-Tracking and Tracking Other(s). But now we add in another level. Noticing what's arising, at the same time, the listener asks herself silently, "What would it be like to be in that situation?" She can approach this in one of two ways:

1. She can connect to a situation in her own life, and remember how she felt. Then she allows herself to re-experience that feeling, and holds that feeling in her body and energy field.

2. Or she can sense into "What would it be like to be the client in this situation? What would it be like to be in his shoes?" Again, the listener then lets herself feel, in her entire body, throughout her body and field, what the client might feel, if he could, if he allowed himself.

3. Now we'll move into the steps of the tool. As the client shares, the listener does the above steps. Now listener—continue to allow yourself to feel as fully as possible. Engage as many senses as possible even as you're listening. Be curious: what's happening physically (any areas of your body tightening? How's your breathing?)

4. What's happening emotionally? Do you want to cry, for example, or do you feel hot with anger? Do you feel scattered and overwhelmed? Do you want to collapse? Do you feel shut down and sleepy?

5. What's happening mentally? What are you thinking about? Is your rational mind cutting off or shutting down your feelings? Are you distracted and thinking about something seemingly unrelated, like what you'll eat soon, or some movie?

6. What's happening spiritually? Is there any belief that you can name that seems related to what the client is describing?

7. Let yourself feel and experience in an embodied way as much as possible whatever you are experiencing.

8. Now hold that feeling, and let it permeate and vibrate through your whole body and energy field. (If this is confusing, think of yourself as like a cello or a double bass. You know how when you hear a cello, you hear that note, and you also "hear-feel" or vibrate with that note, that tone in your body? This is exactly the same. Hold the vibration of what you feel. Or perhaps it helps to think of when you hear the sound of siren

going by outside on the street. Do you know that feeling in your body of hearing with your ears but also "feeling-hearing" the siren, perhaps as a little "shiver" in your body as the sound vibrates through your body and energy field? If this is still confusing, think of tuning forks. When one tuning fork is struck, its tines vibrate and make a sound. The sound waves move through the air. The other tuning fork, which hasn't been struck, harmonically begins to vibrate and makes that same note.

9. If you know that feeling, first hold the vibration of the client's experience in your body and energy field.

10. Now take it a step further. See if you can sense the need underlying that feeling. Ultimately, you don't want to stay vibrationally just like the client. That's the equivalent of jumping into the water along with them if you don't know how to swim, and they don't know how to swim, either. You'll both drown! Instead, now that you vibrationally know what they are experiencing, and have held that state, now see if you can listen for what they need underneath that vibration. What do you sense they are feeling? Angry? Scared? Confused? Happy, but in denial? Genuinely happy?

11. If they are having trouble "dropping into" or connecting with their feelings, and you sense the underlying need, check in with yourself—do you feel willing and able to modulate your field to vibrationally hold the state that they need?

12. For example: If they're angry, do they have a need now to feel loved? If scared, do they have a need now to feel safe? If confused, do they need to feel understood in their confusion, and also clear, meaning, you affirm their ability to make sense of what's confusing? If happy, but in denial, do they need to feel their authentic feelings underlying the denial, or is that too overwhelming right now? If genuinely happy, as with each emotion, is there an underlying need? Maybe, maybe not. Be curious.

13. If you are willing and able, now hold in your own body and field the state needed by the client. You do this by feeling that feeling very strongly in your own body and field. Just like when you "hear-feel" a cello or a siren, now feel the emotional state, what it's like to feel that emotion that they're not letting themselves feel yet, right now.

14. This is not a verbal, mental process. You don't generally mention to the client that you're doing it. You just hold that state vibrationally inside yourself.

15. As you hold the vibration, see if that allows your client to "drop" into what he is feeling. If he is on the "edge" of the feeling, or stuck, does your Resonance allow him to feel his feeling more authentically?

16. As he does feel his feeling more authentically, it will no longer be stuck. It will likely move through him, and he will likely—sometimes quickly—move into the next feeling.

17. Follow his lead, and again meet him where he now is. That is, repeat the steps again. This is one possibility of what may happen.

18. Another possibility is, if he is stuck, he may circle in and out of this "edge."

19. In that case, modulate your energy to come back to meeting him right where he is (the first part of the exercise where you sensed, "What would it be like to be him or 'in his shoes?'"). See if your dropping into the feeling, either in your own life or if you were in his shoes allows him now to really feel it.

20. Keep in mind you are not trying to fix anything. You are not offering suggestions. You are resonating with the feeling, which harmonically gives the client permission to feel whatever he feels. It establishes a safe "field" where he can feel whatever is here now.

21. If appropriate, move into the second part of the tool, where you hold the vibration of the underlying state he may need. See if he drops into his feelings.

22. If instead of dropping, he circles back to his "story" without dropping into his feelings, trust the process: Again, remember that Jung said the psyche has a "gradient towards wholeness," and know this may not be the right time; he may not be ready.

23. Again observe how that is for you. Is that all right with you? Remember you are there to be of service to your client to the best of your ability. You are there to meet the client's needs, not make him be a clone of you or make the same decision you might make or might want to recommend.

24. And it's natural for the needs of the client to evoke feelings in you— that's the nature of relationship. But, again, those feelings in you are not your client's responsibility or problem. You work with your feelings in supervision or with your healer, not with the client.

25. Also keep in mind, as you sense the feeling and/or the need under the feeling, that you may be wrong. That's okay. As you offer a vibrational state by holding that in your own field, you'll quickly get a sense by how

your client responds, as to whether you're on the right track or not. If not, simply adjust. Sometimes even the wrong choice helps the client get clearer on what he is not feeling. So there, as always, your job is not to be perfect, and have everything worked out in your own life already (as if such were even possible). Your job is just to be human and meet a fellow human being right where he is, to the best of your ability.

Chapter Ten
Putting Together Your Practices

Those who have a "why" to live, can bear with almost any "how."

- Viktor Frankl

Putting Together Your Practices

Now let's turn our attention to putting together a plan to meet your needs. You've just learned what you need by using the four tools of the Assessment in the Thriving Through Cancer Method.

Take a look again at your notes on the worksheets from when you worked with each tool. For example, in Self-Tracking, where in your body were you drawn? What did your body let you know you need? If your body didn't want to let you know what you need, then be curious: Might connecting or reconnecting with yourself through your body be your need now?

In Self-Tracking and Tracking Other(s), was anything further revealed to you? Was your healer drawn to the same part of your body as you? Or somewhere else? If somewhere else, did that in any way deepen your experience or provide you with more insight?

What about when you did the Assessment to Foster Discernment? Did you discover that you have further needs, such as the need for more information, the need to know which tests can check if the protocol you're choosing is having an effect? Or did you discover that perhaps you're not using discernment, but rather making decisions based only on your values or beliefs (a very human way to make decisions). And so, realizing that, do you have a need to get comfortable with your choice emotionally, meaning, you know the risks and you're choosing to take them? As an example, as I described in the Prologue, I knew when I learned I have the BRCA1 mutation that I had a high probability of developing both breast and ovarian cancer before age fifty. I could not bring myself to do the prophylactic surgeries. That was a choice based on my values and beliefs—I believed if I developed cancer, we'd catch it early and treat it, and then I'd go on with my life, as my mom has done. That choice was based on feeling that I lived in ways that I believed would make a difference (I was and am a vegetarian; I expressed my feelings, including "negative" emotions like anger, when I felt them; I was very healthy overall.) It was not based on what I now know: that ovarian cancer is not usually cured, as it was with my mom, but instead recurs, some say up to 85% of the time, as we discussed above. Once it comes back, it's considered incurable and ultimately a fatal disease. So I made decisions based on my beliefs, not evidence. But I did decide on surveillance—to do all the testing every six months to detect cancer early if it started. That was a choice based on evidence and advice from the genetic counselor. This is just one example.) Perhaps you, too, are making a choice based solely on your values or beliefs, and by working this skill you discover that you have a need to explain to friends and family that you've made your decision, and now want nothing more than their love and support.

Or, here's a more "getting ready to get ready" version: Do you have a need to begin to consider the possibility that you've been making decisions based solely on your values or beliefs, even if you're not sure yet what you want to do with that awareness? Maybe—like so many of us—you didn't realize your beliefs are how you were basing your decisions. That's extremely common, so common we rarely catch ourselves in the act of making decisions that way.

Here's one more possibility: Did that tool reveal lots of feelings in you about discernment; so now you realize you need support as you talk with someone, and work through your (perhaps conflicting) feelings? These slightly different responses to that tool each highlight unique, but important, needs.

How about Resonance? Did your feelings shift as you talked them through with someone else? Did you "drop" differently than when you worked with the other tools on your own? If so, what was this experience like for you? Do you feel peaceful or all stirred up? What do you need?

Turn now to the worksheet labelled Putting Together Your Practices. Sensing back through your experience as you used the four tools of the

Assessment, what needs became clear or revealed themselves to you? You're looking for physical, emotional, mental and spiritual needs. Sometimes you'll have needs and be aware of them in every area of your life. Other times one or a couple of areas will dominate. Write down anything you noticed.

In the next section, we'll begin to explore specific practices in each of these areas that can help you meet your needs. But first, let's discuss a bit about the practices in general: As with every step of the TTC Method, you can put together and invent practices for yourself. You can also generate and develop a "menu" or "toolkit" of practices in partnership with your client/patient, if you're their healer/therapist/nurse or doctor.

If you're the patient, you can bring the TTC Method to your doctor/therapist/healer, and ask him or her to work the steps with you.

You can work these steps in a group, like a support group. Then you track together what you're doing, work the practices together, and hold each other accountable for showing up and utilizing the practices consistently.

A Couple of Key Points:

1. You can work these tools and practices again and again. Using the Assessment and Practices is meant to be a feedback loop. As you use the practices, your needs will shift, so it's great to familiarize yourself with the full range of practices, so you can then "choose the right tool from the toolbox" based on your current needs, often, quickly and easily.

2. You can track how the practices are working by how you feel, and you can also track by testing. For example, you can see if your symptoms lessen. Lymphedema is a great example. When you get measured for support tights or sleeves, are your limbs smaller because less lymph is stuck and now it's moving through? Or, if you've had surgery and need to regain lung capacity post-op, has the amount of oxygen in your bloodstream increased?

3. I mentioned in the Introduction, and it bears repeating here: I'd love to see research; I'd love studies to be conducted which assess if using this method along with these practices impacts progression-free survival (PFS), overall survival (OS), or "only" or "merely" quality of life.

And as I said, even if this method of assessment and practices "only" affects quality of life, that is a worthwhile benefit. For what is life like if you're not feeling well? If you can feel well, and live normally even as you go through treatment, then your lived experience of life-threatening illnesses like cancer truly feels like you're just living with manageable disease.

Another important note: Do what you can, and when you can't, it's okay. That's also part of tracking your needs. It's important not to forget that, out of some wish to push oneself or be a "good patient" somehow. Another story illustrates this well: In the past, when I was young and healthy, as I described in my story before cancer, I loved to practice ashtanga yoga. If you're familiar with this form, you know it's vigorous, flowing, and helps you develop physical strength (as just one of a slew of benefits far beyond only exercise), quickly. After the "big" surgery, when I had been cut from my pubic bone all the way up to my xiphoid, I had a rough recovery. I was in pain, and weak, but I was also dizzy. A colleague of James' who I'm also friendly with in a professional way talked with me on the phone after that surgery. Trying her best to be helpful, she said, "Jump backs would really help you get your strength back!" (Jump backs are a little like push-ups. You start standing bent forward at the waist with your fingertips touching the floor in front of you. You exhale and put your hands flat on the floor, and then jump your legs backwards, so they end up behind you with your feet flexed, toes touching the floor. You suspend all your body weight in a push-up position between your toes and flat hands.) This colleague meant what she said, and technically, she was right—jump backs do strengthen you. But at that point, I couldn't even remotely do a jump back. I couldn't bend at the waist. I couldn't put my hands down. I could barely walk to the mailbox, and literally needed James to walk backwards while holding my hands. The mailbox was not at our front door, but, in the suburb where we then lived, was a communal hub of metal boxes, all together, up the hill from our house. It was only about a minute-long walk, but every few steps, I'd grab James' hands hard, because I'd get dizzy or winded, and was afraid I'd fall on the cement sidewalk. This did not go away so quickly. Also, at the hospital, the nurse had given me a spirometer to take home and practice with to regain my lung capacity. I'd exhale into it as strongly as I could, but the ball would not go up as high as it should have, in fact had done, just a week earlier, before the surgery. I simply didn't have the breath power.

So, it's a funny story, but this friend's suggestion made me sad, too, because at that point, I was so changed by the operation, I didn't think I'd ever get back to the capabilities I had taken for granted before. So it's important to respect where you actually are, and what your capacity is at any given moment. As you get skilled at using the Assessment tools, you can ask yourself if you want to or can push yourself, and if so, how much, knowing a little bit will likely help you feel better. (As I began to recover, James and I would walk to the mailbox twice a day. Then I could do the walk with a cane. I graduated to walking laps around the house. Then no cane. Jump-backs remained beyond the realm of possibility for quite a while.)

Also keep in mind that the practices give you tools that sometimes solve the same issue as some other practice recommended in conventional medicine (like breathing into the spirometer), but the practice here "multitasks"—it gives you a way "in" to yourself, and so helps you develop your interior sense, rather than just doing a physical exercise by rote.

A Few Notes About the Practices:

As we said at the beginning of Part II, the practices are synergistic. That is, working in each dimension gives you access to all aspects of yourself, and we discussed how the practices are not separated, though I present them that way in this book. In reality, the practices "slide" between physical to emotional to mental to spiritual and any combination of these. Mind-body-spirit connection means we are unified beings.

Let's look at a specific, common example: If you're eating according to how what you eat makes you feel, you'll start to notice that physically of course, but emotionally and mentally as well. Let's look at coffee as an example. Do you notice whether you not only have more energy when you're caffeinated, but you're happier, too? Knowing that, do you want your mood affected, or not? Or how's the crash for you when the caffeine wears off, or when you are not allowed to drink it for some reason? Does this make you want to keep drinking coffee, or stop, or do you not really care? Any answer is okay; the point is that you get to choose.

One of the questions I've always been interested in in terms of this mind-body connection is my sense that mood interacts with cancer. Looking back, I'm aware that in the two years before I was initially diagnosed, I was irritable, angry, and just cranky, often, when earlier in my life, that wasn't so true every day. I asked Steve Cole, PhD, my chicken-and-the-egg question of which comes first, the bad mood or cancer? Dr. Cole is a Professor of Medicine and Psychiatry and Biobehavioral Sciences at UCLA's David Geffen School of Medicine. Using computational bioinformatics, he maps the biological pathways by which social environments influence gene expression by cancer, viral and immune cell genomes.

I first heard Steve discuss gene expression in ovarian cancer as being known now to be affected by perceived social isolation. In other words, if a woman going through ovarian cancer perceives that she is alone and no one around her is there to support her as she goes through it, it doesn't matter if her family and friends really want her to live and will do anything to help make that happen. If, in her mind, she *perceives* that she's alone and isolated, she will recur sooner and metastasize more widely. The latest research now states that this "happens" as the result of gene expression: Genes responsible for recurrence and metastasis "turn on," or "turn off," in response to feelings. This is cutting edge research, as in the past we believed that genes were fixed, immutable; we certainly had no idea that gene expression is affected by emotions.

When I interviewed Dr. Cole for this book, and asked him about persistently being in a bad mood somehow being connected with cancer, he had this to say.

> "It appears to be a two-way street. Cancer, especially before it's detectable as a tumor, is something that would give a feeling of malaise, feeling cruddy, not wanting to spend a lot of time with people you don't know. (And certainly once a tumor grows large enough it causes a feeling of malaise.) Does feeling icky cause cancer? No. Stress doesn't cause cancer. But there is evidence now that stress can make a tumor that's starting and seeded, grow faster, develop blood vessels, metastasize. How? Purely because we evolved that way to handle stress. We evolved to send monocytes to deal with a stress like a cut (invasion of bacteria) or a broken bone. But inadvertently, the cells that we evolved to protect us in these situations (of a hungry beast eating us, for example), while they appeared to help our survival in that situation, inadvertently, accidentally, harm us by making the cancer spread. As the cancer cells liquify, when confronting the monocyte, it allows them to escape and move somewhere else in the body."[17]

So if we're beginning to see evidence that emotional feelings affect gene expression (which you can think about as these switches we mentioned which genes "turn off" and "on"), which in turn affects cancer, it makes sense that as we work with our feelings, that may actually have an effect on cancer. But this is not as simple as telling someone to "think positive" in part, I imagine, because when we enlist our will to try and feel a certain way, that's already a sign that we're not feeling that way; there's actually an underlying, truer feeling. In the case of the woman who perceives she's alone as she goes through ovarian cancer, for example, I imagine that if she just tries to "think positive" she'll still feel alone, and maybe more alone, because even she isn't meeting herself where she really is—by her having a demand that she feel a certain way, she's abandoning herself as well.

Sensing with the body gives you access to the shifting landscape of how you truly feel, moment by moment. Years ago, when I lived in New York, I would go for acupuncture treatments to a Chinese medicine specialist named Ellen Goldsmith. She taught me that emotions equal the flow of energy in the body.

As you work with the practices in the TTC Method, you begin to become aware of the flow of energy. Your observer consciousness watches how what you feel emotionally causes you to make choices. You develop the ability to observe yourself having sensations, and having feelings about body sensations. You draw conclusions and make decisions accordingly. Those emotions cause your body to release hormones or neuropeptides, which increase or decrease sensations, which in turn affect emotions. And the entire cycle repeats.

At the beginning of Part III, we outlined the four tools of the Assessment aspect of the TTC Method before we learned how to work these skills. Under Resonance, we mentioned two scores: the words and tone as one score; and the underlying body language and energy as the other. We talked about how as you listen to someone speak, you can learn to pay attention to the two scores simultaneously—the words they say, and also, at the same time, the feeling and energy underlying the words. Sometimes these will be in agreement, and other times they'll be out of alignment. Both scores are relevant.

This idea of two scores comes from Polish theatre director Jerzy Grotowski. His influence on world theatre was tremendous; starting in the nineteen-sixties, he influenced a whole generation of actors and directors internationally. My MA in his physical approach to actor training was part of how I learned to get out of using only my intellect to live, and instead came to trust in the integration of my mind with my body's ways of knowing.

Grotowski was passionate about exploring with the actors in his troupe what the body can do, without the aid of technology like microphones, lights and gels, masks, and elaborate costumes. He was interested in how to foster the body becoming as expressive as possible. It's his idea that in the most resonant, communicative performances, the actor is performing two, contradictory scores—the words of the play, and the underlying emotions.

One of Grotowski's most famous scenes is in a play called "The Constant Prince," in which he directed his star male actor, Ryszard Cieslak, to perform playing two simultaneous scores. First there were the lines of the play, the words Cieslak said, that the audience heard. Grotowksi's work is influenced by the fact that he was a child in (Catholic) Poland during the Second World War. The play concerns Jesus' dying as a martyr for people's sins, and Cieslak inhabited that aspect of the role convincingly: He was pale, thin, and naked but for his costume of only a loincloth. At the same time, Grotowski directed Cieslak to, with his body, enact the first time he ever made love. The way he moved his hands, his arms, his pelvis, his head, his mouth, when he closed his eyes—he was depicting lovemaking. Even as the words he spoke had to do with suffering and martyring himself, the physical actions depicted quite a different passion.

It's similar with these practices: there's the overt aim of them (for example, to get strong after surgery, or to feel as well as possible as you undergo chemo), but then there's the other score—not only to rebuild your strength, but to develop a sense of yourself from your interior, from the inside out, so that you know how you are, you know what you can do; you deepen connection with yourself even as you go through treatment and recovery.

It is this deep self-connection that I suspect someday we will know promotes rehabilitation and aids survival.

In Part I, I described my experience with cancer, and in Part II, described how everything in my life before I knew there were other options, kept me up in my head, or outside myself, caught in the exterior, wrapped up in others' perceptions both of me and of life in general. Before I knew about energy healing, like so many of us today, I was smart, but not embodied. As I've described, it's been a long process of coming home to a vital, shifting, interior sense of myself.

But once a person comes to a sense of integration, it is recognizable. We know it in each other when we have senses to perceive it. For example, I first began to practice grounding and filling myself with energy every day when I started studying at the healing school. Where I had been too skinny before and each ride standing on the subway meant I'd be swept off balance by every screeching stop or start of the train, as I began practicing, I effortlessly got to a normal weight and could stand on the moving train without holding on to any support and without losing my balance. I remember one teacher at the school retired, and when he came to visit the following year, we bumped into each other in the hallway. "Wow, you look different!" he said. He said he could tell I was more present, more embodied.

Similarly, but in a different context, just a few years ago, when James and I were first considering immigrating to the Netherlands, I called several potential immigration attorneys. As I described how James and I are each self-employed, and the seminars and workshops I planned to teach in Amsterdam, I mentioned the particular historic hotel where I had looked into hosting future workshops. With one lawyer in particular, as I elaborated the specifics of how and why I love Amsterdam, and how I would love to teach here, I noticed a softening in his energy and voice as we discussed potential business structures I could set up for me to live and work here legally. The words were likely the same, but it was as though he could tell I was serious about immigrating and had done the legwork, but he could also sense my love for his home. Though still a business call, he softened, and I could tell he warmed to me. And he could tell that I could tell, and so the whole conversation became delicious. This is what embodiment looks, sounds, and feels like. The benefits are applicable and apparent in every situation.

I think Viktor Frankl meant something similar when he wrote, "A human being is a deciding being." He survived life in concentration camps in the Second World War. Afterwards, he described how yes, he had to endure life in the camps. But the Nazis could not take from him his inner state. They could not control what he thought and felt inside. And he realized that love was the most important feeling. He could not change the fact of suffering. But he could change himself inside.

Similarly, with this Method and these practices, you get to decide how you feel. You can, if you choose, learn how to manage your own inner state most of the time. If you choose to connect with yourself even as you go through grueling medical procedures, you can brave the experiences, and feel empowered, more resilient, rather than "felled" by the medical ordeals.

Then ordinary life feels exquisite, even if and as we undergo suffering. And the times of not suffering—for example after cancer, when you're well again—these can feel even richer than before.

CHAPTER ELEVEN
PHYSICAL PRACTICES

That summer there was no girl left in me.
It gradually became clear.
It suddenly became.

In the pool, I was more heavy than light.
Pockmarked and flabby in a floppy hat.
What will my body be

When parked all night in the earth?
Midsummer. Breathe in. Breathe out.
I am not on the oxygen tank.

Twice a week we have sex.
The lithe girls poolside I see them
at their weddings I see them with babies their hips

thickening I see them middle-aged.
I can't see past the point where I am.
Like you, I'm just passing through.

I want to hold on awhile.
Don't want to naught
or forsake, don't want

To be laid gently or racked raw.
If I retinol. If I marathon.
If I Vitamin C. If I crimson
my lips and streakish my hair.
If I wax. Exfoliate. Copulate
beside the fish-slicked sea.

Fill me I'm cold. Fill me I'm halfway gone.
Would you crush me in the stairwell?
Could we just lie down?

If the brakes don't work.
If the pesticides won't wash off.
If the seventh floor pushes a brick

out the window and it lands on my head.
If a tremor, menopause. Cancer. ALS.
These are the ABCs of my fear.

The doctor says
I don't have a pill for that, dear.
Well, what would be a cure-all, ladies,

gin-and-tonics on a summer night?
See you in the immortalities! O blurred.
O tumble-rush of days we cannot catch.

- Deborah Landau, "Solitaire"

Unify Your Mind and Body and Physical Practices

Now as we move into the section on the practices themselves of the Thriving Through Cancer Method, you're going to make a personalized toolkit of the practices that meet your needs that you can then use. As you work the practices, you'll then assess again (using the four tools of the Assessment that you just learned in that section, above). As you reassess, you'll see which needs you've met, which remain, and which have shifted, so now call for some new practice to meet your current need. Then you'll choose new practices, work those, and repeat. Thus you can feel better and better, more whole, no matter what's going on in your life.

Now as you read through the physical, emotional, mental and spiritual practices, make notes on your worksheet (the one you were just working with, "Putting Together Your Practices"), of which ones appeal to you. Consider it like thumbing through a cookbook; let what appeals to you be your guide. Before you know it, you've planned a multi-course meal. If you make all the dishes, soon those yummy courses become memorable, more than if you just cook one entree. All together, they make a feast.

So we're going to start with the Physical Practices, and this all sounds great, but as I start to write about all these ways to come back into contact with oneself physically, my resistance increases. I keep hopping up to grab a snack. Then I want hand cream; my skin feels dry. Next I want to look at Facebook. After that, I'm restless. Why? What's going on?

This is an example of what I described above about why we need this Method—how, if we let it, the world can be distractive. The truth is, for me, the Physical Practices transform my state fast. When I'm cranky, there's nothing that helps me feel blissful as quickly as if I exercise in some quiet, internally-focused way. Yet although I know that, even after all these years, it's still a silent argument I have with myself regularly, about whether I'll give myself permission to spend time doing what I love. Can you relate?

I also think for many of us alive today there's another factor: Being this embodied feels slow and inefficient. There's not much reward in our society for being deliberately unproductive. It's acceptable only at certain times, for example when we get a manicure. That can feel relaxing, and it's condoned as an acceptable means of self-soothing by certain classes, but it doesn't help us connect to our interior.

Let's think about it another way: Our bodies are so vulnerable. They are the locus where struggles get enacted—politically, environmentally, in intimate relationships, in wars, and of course in disease. Another way of saying this is the body is a microcosm of the world. The old Hermetic idea of "As above, so below," might also be understood as "As outside," (externally, in the world), "so inside" (internally, even to the level of the cell, for example).

All the religions of the world recognize the power of the body to evoke feelings and behavior, and so legislate about how to manage all that our bodies arouse in us. In case you think this is too abstract, consider the recent "burkini" ban in France. (A burkini is a word made by combining the words "burka" and "bikini." It is lightweight clothing made for women to wear while swimming, and it is said to go along with the Islamic traditions of modest dress. It covers the entire body except for the face, hands and feet. Women in France in summer 2016 were suddenly told it was illegal for them to wear the burkini; they were fined if they wore one. At the same time, the Muslim religion believes in both males and females dressing "modestly," and there are various ways women dress "modestly," including by wearing the niqab (a veil which covers the head and face, just leaving the eyes showing). It is usually worn with an abaya (a robe) that covers the body from head to feet. Women might also wear a hijab (covers the hair and neck, but not the face), or a burka (which covers the entire face and body, with a mesh window in front of the eyes to see through).

Islam is not the only religion that legislates about the body. Religious Jewish men cover their heads with a kippah, also called a yarmulke. Married religious Jewish women are required to immerse themselves in a mikveh, a private, ritual bath, to sanctify her after each month's menstruation and after giving birth to a child.

The Holy Communion of Christianity is a rite said to be given by Jesus to his disciples at the Last Supper, where he commanded them to eat the bread as his "body," and drink the wine as his "blood," and to do so in memory of him—to remember his upcoming crucifixion as his sacrifice and martyrdom.

These are religious examples, but look at any news report, and, all over the world, the headlines are about the body, and not just what the body awakens, but about the body itself. Lately the stories concern civilians in Aleppo, Syria trying to survive the war that they are not fighting, just stranded in. Parts of the city have no water, and aid convoys keep being bombed. Refugees have walked or tried to come by boat from the Middle East and also from Somalia to Europe; it's the largest exodus of refugees since the Second World War. Many have drowned in the Mediterranean and not made it. In the US, there is a crisis with police shooting unarmed Black men, and in general, people shooting each other with guns. What do these news items have in common? The body. None of these issues is philosophical to the people living through these experiences. These are not merely hypothetical, intellectual policy debates, and they are not only about emotions. These are life and death struggles playing out in our vulnerable human bodies, in fact using our human bodies to affect ideas about how life should be.

These are examples from contemporary politics and history. And if you read this book far in the future when these issues have passed, there will almost certainly be the matters of your day, which are the same issues. Every war in history has been about the vulnerability of human bodies and what we do to each other.

Consider popular culture. So many movies lately depict a world where humans are somehow in battle with armies that are super-human or not human, and thus seemingly invincible. People become "superheroes" with attributes that make them more—better than—human. But underneath, each character has an all too human flaw that leaves that character open to attack. What makes these stories compelling is that against all odds, the exposed humans, with our human bodies, triumph. We can look at "Star Wars," with its battle between the Shadow, personified by Darth Vader, Kylo Ren, the Siths, etcetera, and those who must use the light side of "the Force" in their human ability to commune with the coherent universe, and yet are vulnerable because of being human. Or take "District 9," where man in all his arrogance, through a cocky attempt to dominate the aliens living in the midst of their society, has an accident that causes the aliens' DNA to blend with the protagonist's. In the process, he loses everyone he loves and all aspects of human life; ultimately, he becomes alien, and so is ostracized in the true sense of the word, banished in a way that jeopardizes his very survival.

Even the recent phenomenon of Internet "trolling," where people attack each other and hurl verbal and emotional abuse at each other through hostile online posts, may seem at first glance to be different because of its anonymity. It becomes a trend we discuss however, when it leads to a level of bullying that causes suicide—again, each time the death of someone real, a specific, not anonymous, living person, not an avatar.

Seen from this perspective, we see that the human race is caught up in a many centuries-long obsession about the possibilities and limits of what it means to be alive in a human body.

Our discussions about the singularity and artificial intelligence are part of the same pattern. What interests us is: Will we be dominated by the machines we create? Or will we outpace death and live forever in an (albeit false) belief that we can fully control our lives in these human bodies?

These questions take us back to Descartes' idea that the body is a machine that can be reduced to its parts; like a clock, it can be taken apart and put back together again. He believed all reality that can be experienced is either "spatial" or "conscious being or existence." In Descartes' worldview, spatial (the quality of filling space, that is our corporeality, our qualities of existing inside bodies), and consciousness ("extension" and "thought") are the simplest, original, and the only two attributes of reality, and these two are divided. Something can be either spatial or consciousness, body or mind, but not both.[18]

Descartes lived in the Netherlands for more than twenty years, first in 1618 as a young soldier, then again starting in 1628. In Amsterdam, he lived near where James and I love to go eat the best apple pie in the city. Amsterdam at that time was a hotbed of religious debate and scientific exploration. It was a center of publishing, and then, as today, a very international, cosmopolitan, yet intimate, village-like place.

Living in Amsterdam, as I now do, I can imagine Descartes walking these same streets, mulling over his ideas. The Waag, or weigh house, where the famous Rembrandt painting that depicts the Amsterdam surgeons looking on as a public dissection of a man's arm takes place—that building is five minutes from our apartment; I pass it on my bike nearly every day.

Yet that painting, "The Anatomy Lesson of Dr. Nicolaes Tulp" which is considered so emblematic of its time, illustrates the problem with Descartes' dualism. The painting was painted by a twenty-six year old, newly arrived in the city, Rembrandt, likely when Descartes had also just moved back here after graduating from Leiden University,

The painting depicts a unique person, the criminal Aris Kindt—who was convicted of armed robbery and sentenced to death by hanging. He had been executed earlier that day, January 31, 1632. There he lies, the autopsy underway, his left arm dissected, the anatomy textbook propped open at his feet. Dr. Tulp, the city's Anatomist, is seen explaining the musculature of Kindt's arm. The members of the surgeons' guild are seen looking on, and again, they are specific men, and they, along with Dr. Tulp, paid to be depicted in the portrait. The painting was hung in the Waag building, where the surgeons had their guild office, and where the dissection took place, both in real life and in the artwork.

Besides the history and the specificity—here we are, watching the early days of science, in a building that still stands and is now a restaurant, with people who look not so different from the Dutch hipsters of today with their van Dyke beards—besides all that, what we see depicted are the men's feelings about seeing inside another man's arm. Several lean forward, they furrow their brows, they stare; they're curious and want to know the truth. But exactly there, in that painting, is the holistic mind-body unity that Rembrandt is famous for and that Descartes sought to bifurcate. Rembrandt captures the inner state of the people whose portraits he painted. Right there we see what we all experience—we see the body of the dead man, and we see the feelings of the people as they watch. We are more than merely spatial or consciousness. We are both.

We all know this. We recognize it when we see it. Three years after this painting, Descartes became a father. Five years after that, his daughter died, and Descartes is known to have cried.[19]

We can attempt to reduce our experience in any number of ways (our emotions are merely chemical or hormonal, as one example), but the notion that we should explain complex phenomena by the simplest possible underlying principles in order to get to the truth, does not agree with our lived, interior experience. By simplifying matters, we lose the mind-body holistic connections, which agree with our perceptions if only we let them.

So now, as we begin the Physical Practices, keep in mind that this is what we're going for—the delicious fullness of the feast we talked about at the beginning of this chapter, the empirical knowing that the whole is greater than the sum of the parts.

If, as Descartes believed, we are clocks that can be dismantled and reassembled, then we are also the carving of the wood into the shape of the cabin that houses the mechanism, as well as the hand that held the knife—the maker who coaxed the wood we are into that clock. We are the paintings of the sun and the moon on the clock face that give so much delight, as they emerge and disappear every twenty-four hours. We are the cuckoo that bursts forth and chirps to count each hour, before disappearing again behind the tiny wooden door, back into the birdhouse when the counting is complete, until the next hour when the bird will, like clockwork, sing to count the hours again.

CHAPTER TWELVE
PHYSICAL MOVEMENT PRACTICES

Stop acting so small. You are the universe in ecstatic motion.

\- Jalaluddin Rumi

Physical Movement Practices

So now as we move into the physical practices, keep in mind that everything you do, you do to develop this mind-body unity and where we understand it with biochemical proof already, to work in conjunction with that interconnection. When you dance, you dance from how it feels, how your body wants to move, rather than how it looks from the outside watching you dance.

When you use your voice, you use it from how it feels to make different sounds with your lips and your breath moving through your lungs and out through the resonators in certain chakras (which we'll define and learn about below).

When you eat, you choose what to eat to affect your bioterrain, your interior environment on the cellular level, which affects how you feel. David Servan-Schreiber, MD, PhD, a doctor who had brain cancer, wrote *Anticancer*. There he puts forth a diet to affect one's bioterrain, that is, the inner "microclimate" of the cells, and thus to potentially improve one's chances of survival. Because he was a doctor, and he cited legitimate research, MD Anderson partnered with him to study and bolster complementary cancer care.

Similarly, the Block Center for Integrative Cancer Treatment, founded by Keith Block, MD, teaches patients how to eat to affect bioterrain to make a less hospitable environment for cancer cells. Block also brought chronomodulated chemotherapy to his center in Illinois, as one of only a handful of US treatment centers to offer it. Yet, according to Block, forty major centers in Europe participate in cooperative research using time-based protocols for chemo administration because that is more effective and beneficial for patients. Working with the "clock-related genes" that control time-dependent biological functions, including eating and sleeping patterns, body temperature, heart rate, and hormone production, researchers have found that normal cells and cancer cells have different times when they rest and divide. By giving chemotherapy at the time when it will have the greatest effect on cancer cells, and less toxic effects on healthy cells, Block claims he's been able to reduce side effects and improve survival.[20]

With exercise, we know that moving our bodies increases survival. Dr. Asher, at Cedars-Sinai in Los Angeles (the doctor we mentioned above in connection with his program for small groups of people dealing with advanced stage cancer), also runs an exercise program for people after they've survived cancer. He had this to say about physical activity, and he touched on the survival benefits that we know about, and those we see but don't yet know how to explain:

> "Exercise is so untapped in using it as a meaningful intervention. There was a recent study of women with metastatic breast cancer. They found that your fitness level, how cardiovascularly in shape you are, clearly affects survival. It improves fatigue and survival, and the social aspect is also therapeutic. Even in women with metastatic cancer: They age twenty to thirty years by having cancer, but this can be mitigated by exercise. Exercise helps with depression, sleep, reducing inflammatory mediators. Tumors may feed off inflammatory chemicals. Reducing body fat? Exercise does this. There's less estrogen because fat can make estrogen. And the idea that insulin maybe feeds cancers? When you're not in shape, you have insulin resistance and need to produce more insulin. So we know

this about exercise. But there are many things we don't know. Even women with breast cancer that is estrogen receptor negative still have survival benefits."[21]

This to me highlights the possibility that there appear to be benefits to harnessing a connection between one's body and mind that we do not completely understand yet, though we see evidence which hints that it may be important.

Dr. Friedman, the surgeon, demystified it. When I interviewed him for the book, he talked about my case in particular to illustrate his points. He said, "When we see somebody like you, we know we can get away with whatever surgery we need to do, and treat aggressively. We don't know if we'll win, but we can be *aggressive.*"[22] I know when going through cancer, I treated exercise as though I were in training for some big event, like a marathon. Not to say that I trained that hard, but I treated exercise as something I needed to do every day if possible, so I could live as long as possible. Dr. Friedman implied that "you may not be able to take so many actions once you're diagnosed," but I disagree. I feel like exercising—obviously while respecting where you are and how you're feeling and what you're able to do—can actually help you develop greater health, even as you go through treatment.

The key here is not simply to exercise mindlessly, but rather, it's important when you exercise to do so "from the inside out." Remember my story of not being able to get the ball to go as high as it should when I practiced breathing exercises with the spirometer after the "big surgery"? What you're about to learn is completely different than that.

So as we move into the first physical practice, keep in mind that we're going for is moving from how it feels rather than how it looks. Every practice helps you come back home to yourself, each in a different way.

Movement from How it Feels Rather Than How it Looks

As with all the practices, first take a baseline reading of where you are right now. If you'd like, you can refer again to the worksheet, "Your Baseline Before Self-Tracking" to recall the steps. Essentially, you want to always get a sense of where you are before you do any practice, and then take a baseline reading again after you've done the practice to notice what has shifted.

So, quickly scan through your body now, and notice how your breathing is (shallow? Or deep?). Notice any areas of physical pain or tension and where these are. Pay attention to what mood you're in, how you're feeling emotionally. Observe what you're thinking about. Perceive how you're feeling spiritually, which may be as simple as feeling unified and connected, or not. As always, there are no right or wrong answers here, you're just getting a sense of how you are right in this moment.

1. Now that you've taken your baseline, we'll start this movement practice. If you're not yet standing up, stand up now. Look around the room so you know how much space you have in which to move, and what's nearby. You want to avoid bumping into anything because you'll be moving with your eyes closed. (Once this practice is familiar to you, you don't have to start standing up; you can start from any position, sitting on a chair, lying down on the floor, etcetera. But for now, start standing.)

2. Let your gaze soften, and then close your eyes.

3. First notice: What happens inside you as you close your eyes? Does anything shift from not being able to see? How's your breathing? How's your heart rate?

4. Start to go inside more now. Start moving from how it feels rather than how it looks.

5. (If you're doing this with a group and you don't know each other well yet, or haven't practiced this a lot together, start with your eyes open, but with a soft gaze. Look three feet (about one meter) diagonally forward in front of you so you see the floor. This will allow you to go into deep contact with yourself, but also notice if someone is so near you you might bump into each other. (Once you're more familiar with this practice, you'll be able to keep your eyes closed in a group and sense how close you are from others with your dorsal spine. This is apparently a residual ability left from ontogeny recapitulating phylogeny, the theory that we, in developing from embryo to adult (ontogeny), contain all the stages of evolution (phylogeny). It's a fascinating theory, out of favor nowadays, but surprisingly easy to experience this part of it: that we can each somehow sense distance with our dorsal spine.)[23]

6. Now ask: Which part of your body would like to move first? Let that part initiate movement. For example, does your elbow feel like moving

first? Then let your elbow start. Which way does it want to move? How far? See if at the full range of motion, your elbow wants to extend all way from your elbow, to your forearm, hand, fingers?

7. What happens next? Do you want to move your elbow in a different direction? Or another body part?

8. You're not thinking about how it looks or worrying "How's my dancing?"

9. Instead, you're beginning to hone your proprioceptive sense, your ability to sense from inside your body and what your body wants, how you want to move.

10. As you consider this, now add in the quality to your movement that your body wants: How do you want to move? Slowly? Arcing? Gracefully? Fast? Staccato? Strongly?

11. Now add in *gestures*: Do you feel like poking? Thrusting? Sliding? Floating?

12. Great. Now ask, what *tempo* do you want to move at now? Fast or slow? Move that speed. Change when you notice you want to change.

13. Now we're going to deepen further: Notice if part of your body moves, while another part remains frozen. For example, do you enjoy moving your head, and find your head naturally moves, but your pelvis doesn't?

14. Be curious: What makes you enjoy moving some parts of your body and not others? As always, there's no wrong or right answer. There's no superego voice saying you "should" move any frozen parts. Just be curious.

15. So, what's it like to move through space? Are you staying near where you started? Or moving throughout the available space? Or somewhat in between these two—are you moving a little bit? Notice: Is this familiar? Ask yourself: Do you tend to be cautious? Or brash?

16. What happens inside when I ask you that? Just notice.

17. So this is your dance. It's all about you. Not about relating to others or interacting with a dance partner. It's not about merging with music. It's all about where you are, right now. So this internally-focused movement is one of the physical practices in the TTC Method. It's different from traditional exercise and almost every style of dance because of this focus inside. Imagine how a few minutes of this can help you come back into contact with yourself.

18. Picture a patient recovering from surgery: Perhaps she's supposed to walk laps around the hospital wing she's in and practice breathing with the spirometer, like in my story. Those are great ways to get your strength back. But they're different; they don't have this focus on your interior.

19. I developed this method as an outgrowth of my theatre and dance training. And this way of moving may be too much at the beginning. That's okay. But you can adapt this practice. You can go inside even from a hospital bed—you can envision yourself moving even if you can't do it right now, or can't do it yet. Many athletes "rehearse" in their minds how specifically to compete at whatever their sport is. They are not moving at all at these moments, but it's a key part of their preparation to be their most competitive.

20. For you, you can break this exercise down as much as you need. You can go inside a little bit as you sit on the edge of your bed with your feet touching the floor. Working with this practice will help you know when you want to move, and when you don't. It can help you get used to the "new normal" of "this is my body right now, post-op/post-treatment."

21. And while there may be sadness for how your body right now can't do certain movements that you may have taken for granted in the past, still, by being with what is, right here, right now, there's also the possibility that you might feel righteous, like, "I survived the surgery. Here I am." And by moving, even in these perhaps small ways, your body can find the way "home" to you again.

22. So now take a baseline reading again, a quick body scan. How are you now? Do you sense this quality of coming home to yourself by moving this way? If so, how is that for you? If not, what's coming up for you?

Sue Hitzmann's MELT Method

So far we've looked at the physical practice of movement from how it feels rather than how it looks. I've said this focus on how it feels is a vital key to develop an interior sense of yourself. I now want to recommend the specific practice I mentioned in sharing my story of going through cancer, above; this not part of the TTC Method, but it complements everything I teach here. Sue Hitzmann's MELT Method—which is an easy way to rehydrate your fascia using her patented foam rollers and small balls—has had such a profound effect on my life and health that I highly recommend it.

Particularly if you have lymphedema, pain, dizziness, or balance issues, the MELT Method is a simple, quick to do, easy to learn way for you to feel better right away.

When I went to my first MELT Method session in 2015, I had constant symptoms of lymphedema in both my legs. My legs were swollen from my ankles all the way up to my groin and they felt heavy and looked big from all the lymph that wasn't moving. This problem had started after the second-look surgery in 2012, when I had some fourteen inguinal lymph nodes removed from my groin. While I was told before that surgery "lymphedema won't happen to you," and afterwards that my case was "not severe," still, I was prescribed the tights with forty pounds of pressure on each leg, the strongest amount of compression available. These inelegant, thick, black nylon thigh-highs squeezed in a graduated way up each leg so the lymph could move up into my pelvis, where I still had lymph nodes, and they could do the work of filtering cellular waste products from my body. Without the tights, I felt like I was walking underwater in wet jeans. It was uncomfortable. Wearing the tights, I looked chubby, and could see the elastic bands at the top of each stocking around my thighs through my jeans. I wore green rubber gloves to get those tights on and off, and getting dressed took an extra fifteen minutes every morning.

This went on every day for three years. My shoes were all a half size larger. My watch even needed to be worn on a looser hole in the band. I was swollen all over.

Then my "California Mom," my mother-in-law, Dee, recommended I try MELT Method. She had been practicing for a few years with excellent results. Her trainer at her gym taught her, so I, too, became a pupil of Gloria Stewart.

Gloria is extremely good at this proprioceptive sensing we've been describing. Her way of listening with her body sense is highly attuned, and she knew how to watch me exercise and put her fingertip or hand right where I needed it to teach me how to move in a way that would help me feel better.

Gloria is one of Sue Hitzmann's MELT Master Trainers. There are currently six in the world, and Gloria is one of them. As I began to practice MELT Method, I noticed changes right away. At first, I just felt less dizzy, like my right and left sides came back into sync. Then I could breathe deeply again, even where there is scar tissue from my diaphragm having been "stripped." After a while, my legs stopped swelling. Now if I practice regularly, I no longer need to wear the tights. (I still wear them when I fly on planes, but not every day anymore.) This is a huge improvement. If I don't practice for a few days, the swelling starts to come back, so MELT Method hasn't cured me, but it's transformed my experience. I've gone back to my regular shoe size and my watchband is back to my size.

So this is an example of how you can use what you notice from the Assessment where you learn your needs (which I'm sure you can hear in my description of all the ways the lymphedema symptoms cramped my style), and then look for and implement solutions.

Now when I go to doctor's appointments and see other women in the waiting rooms who have lymphedema (and they have it severely, to the point where young survivors of their cancers can't walk unassisted, or they can't easily fit in a chair, or their ankles swell over their feet), I feel both enraged and like there are "things" that can help. I feel angry because I can see the problem is far more common than that surgeon led me to believe when he said, with a wink, it wouldn't happen to me. But I feel like the promise of this era is that we can share information. MELT Method works very well for me, and I am so grateful to Gloria, for teaching it to me, Dee, for recommending it, and to Sue Hitzmann for developing it.

CHAPTER THIRTEEN
PHYSICAL-ENERGETIC PRACTICES

*Discovery consists of seeing what everybody has seen
and thinking what nobody has thought.*

- Albert von Szent Gyorgy

Chakra System, Hara, Inner Light, Voicework

The Chakra System

The chakra system is a map of where subtle energy overlays, enters, interacts with and affects the physical human body. It is also a map of human psycho-spiritual development.

The word chakra means "wheel" in Sanskrit, and it is believed that we humans have these chakras, or wheels, in specific locations in our bodies. The turning of these chakras brings energy into our bodies from the world around us (if they're turning clockwise), and depletes our bodies of energy (if they're turning counterclockwise). Keep in mind our definition of health as the energy flowing, and disease as the blockage or weakening of the flow of energy, and you can see the origin of that definition in this conception of the chakras. Another way of saying our chakras are turning clockwise is to describe them as "open," and when our chakras are open, we get charged with energy as we go about our daily activities. Our chakras are closed (meaning turning counterclockwise) when we are not well or are in emotional defense. When they are still, they do not rotate at all, and no energy moves.

There are seven main chakras. These wheels are metaphorical: it is not as though if someone died and an autopsy were conducted, we would find literal wheels inside the body.

Instead, everywhere where there is a chakra, that place corresponds to a plexus of nerve endings that emanate from the spinal column. Essentially, the chakra system is the Ayurvedic depiction (Ayurveda being the medical system of India), of what in Western medicine is called the endocrine system.

With one important distinction: The chakra system also includes an understanding of human development. We humans are said to ascend a progressive "ladder" of requirements needed to be human, much like Maslow's hierarchy of needs. The bottom rung of the ladder starts with the concerns of the first chakra, that is, elements necessary for basic survival—food, shelter, clothing, safety—and each step builds on its predecessor, ultimately rising to a sense of cosmic spiritual oneness (the realm of the seventh chakra).

Some say that the Staff of Asclepius, the symbol of medicine in ancient Greece (one snake twisting around and up a central pole), and the caduceus (the familiar two snakes who both twist and cross up a central pole, ending with wings at the top, and often used to represent the medical profession in the West), are cross-cultural representations of the chakra system—everywhere the snakes cross each other and the staff is said to be like a chakra whose tips touch into the central "pole" of our spinal cord.

There's a similar representation in kundalini yoga, in which there are said to be two "snakes" of energy, called Ida and Pingala, coiled at the base of the spine. As the snakes awaken and ascend the sushumna (central column, like the spinal cord in the West), we humans develop from survival to a sense of spiritual unity.

The chakras are mentioned in the Vedas, the oldest written literature in India (1500-500 BC), which are collected from earlier oral tradition. The Upanishads (circa 600 BC) and the yoga sutras of Patanjali (circa 200 BC) also mention the chakras.

You can use the chakra system as a way to understand the progression of your own personal, human development on every level—physically, emotionally, mentally and spiritually. As a set of guideposts, the chakra system can help you come to know where you might be having issues in life, by trying to "skip ahead," and ignoring certain aspects of life. (For example, do you love to meditate and practice yoga, but find buying groceries or even the need to eat all the time boring? Is it challenging to balance your checkbook or even focus on how to earn money? These issues might indicate you're developing your spiritual side (represented by your seventh chakra), but trying to circumvent ordinary, daily life (represented by your first).

Energetically, the chakra system can also serve as a map to notice where your energy is flowing (and thus you are healthy), and where it is blocked (so where you might be feeling dis-eased). Based on what you sense, you can work practices to keep your chakras charged, balanced, and clear.

Remember how I mentioned that before healing school I was ungrounded, but how as I began to practice daily, I could ride the subway without holding on to any support? I used chakra-opening practices, among others, to keep my energy field clear, strong and balanced. But when I left the healing school, and went through that crisis of belief in my modality, I stopped working with those practices. These words don't convey the depth of my disappointment—it was more like I completely abandoned the practices that I had loved, and that had sustained me. By that I mean, I forsook myself. It's an old-fashioned word, but that's how I felt—like I renounced what was most dear to me. This went on for about two years—no daily chakra opening, no sensing to see how I was doing energetically. I didn't next check my chakras until I was literally on the gurney, wearing nothing but a scratchy green hospital gown and a thick, fibrous paper hairnet covering my hair to keep everything sterile, my glasses not in front of my eyes, but removed by the orderly, and given to James to hold, as I was being wheeled down the long hallways of the hospital, on the way to the operating room, into that first surgery. Could I have waited any longer?

On that ride, when I desperately tried to open my chakras (which we'll discuss how you, too, can do, just below), it was immediately clear to me that my first and second chakras were not open, and by keeping them closed, I had been cutting myself off from any connection to the earth. I had gone back to being ungrounded. This was my old habit, and I was shocked that I had reverted to this way of "running my energy" so quickly, completely, and automatically. I felt so sad, and had a feeling at that moment that I was not well; and I won't go so far as to say I was not well because I had betrayed myself, but my self-abandonment did feel like a key factor. (This is not to blame myself. I am not saying I "caused" the cancer or that that is even possible. I am saying I felt disconnected from myself, and all that I know nourishes me. I know I was doing the best I could at the time, but it was confirmed to me again in that moment that energy is real, and palpable, and I had been willfully denying my empirical evidence of that, for a long time.)

For you, if this is a new tool, you'll find it's useful as a quick way to see how you are running your energy at any given moment. You can use the practice in two ways: One, to assess how your energy is flowing. Two, you can also use it to feel better. If you're experiencing fatigue, pain, feeling cut off from yourself, worried, afraid, or angry, then focusing on breathing into each chakra and opening it can relieve stress, get the energy moving again, and help you feel like you can focus on something else other than whatever you're worried about; it can be an act of self-love.

Just below, we'll move into a description of each chakra. You can work with your chakra system in several ways:

1. You can breathe into every chakra and direct your attention to each one, sequentially;

2. You can look at something—an article of clothing or piece of fabric, paper, a paint chip— that is that chakra's color, and let your eyes and body "drink in" that color (literally, that frequency of energy).

3. You can make the corresponding sound or note of that chakra's frequency.

4. You can "see" the color by picturing it in your mind's eye. In other words, you enlist your senses of hearing, seeing, feeling, smelling, tasting, and/or just knowing to fill your body and field with energy.

The results of having and keeping your chakras clear, balanced, and charged are:

1. You have a healthy flow of energy.

2. Issues to do with your personality concerns have more flow. By that I mean you can become less defended, more open, less self-protective, and more curious about others, while at the same time being in contact with yourself.

Here Are the Seven Chakras:

1. The first chakra, or root chakra, is known in Sanskrit as the Muladhara chakra. It is located at the base of the spine. It is red. The "bija mantra" or "seed mantra," that is, the sound you can make with your voice to vibrate at the same frequency as this chakra, is "lam." The musical note is C. Its symbol is a square. It is connected to the adrenal glands, the rectum, the elimination system, hips, legs, feet, and the spine. The first chakra concerns basic survival needs like food, shelter, clothing, connection with the earth, your tribe, and family. To keep your first chakra open, you can hike, walk barefoot in nature, dance, especially

dance styles which emphasize connection with the earth, with lots of contact specifically between your feet and the ground, and movements like stomping rhythmically, such as in African dance.

2. The second chakra, or sacral chakra, in Sanskrit is known as the Svadhishthana chakra. It is located in the middle of the pelvis, and corresponds to the whole reproductive system and specifically the ovaries in females and testes in males. The color of the second chakra is orange, and the corresponding seed mantra is "vam." The musical note is D. Its symbol is an upturned crescent. The second chakra concerns sexuality, fertility, creativity, and feelings about yourself. To keep your second chakra open you can do styles of dance that emphasize the pelvis, such as belly dancing. You can make love. You can move your pelvis.

3. The third chakra or solar plexus chakra, in Sanskrit is the Manipura chakra. It is right where your ribs separate. The corresponding seed mantra is "ram," its note is E, and its symbol is a descending triangle. The color associated with this chakra is yellow. It is the place of your "gut feelings," your sense of yourself in the world. It corresponds to the stomach, pancreas, liver, spleen, gallbladder and digestive system. You can practice deep breathing to keep this chakra open. You can put your hands on your belly, and then on the sides of your ribs to sense this deep way of breathing.

4. The fourth chakra or heart chakra is the Anahata chakra in Sanskrit. The color is green, and the seed mantra is "yam." The note is F-sharp. The symbol of the fourth chakra is intertwined descending and ascending triangles—a six-pointed star. It is right between your breasts, whether you are female or male. The fourth chakra corresponds to the thymus, heart, lungs, breasts, as well as the circulatory system, and the respiratory system. It is all about love. It is the bridge between the lower three and upper three chakras, between the concerns of ordinary life as represented in chakras one, two, and three, and our bond with Spirit, however you understand that tie for yourself, in the upper three chakras (five, six, and seven). A practice to keep your heart chakra open is to think of someone you love. Hugging also keeps the heart chakra healthy. Any kind of cardiovascular exercise is great for the heart chakra.

5. The fifth chakra or throat chakra: Called the Vishuddha chakra in Sanskrit, the color is sky blue, and its seed mantra is "hum." The note is G. The symbol of the fifth chakra is a circle within a descending triangle. It corresponds to the thyroid, parathyroid, the throat, larynx, esophagus,

and the neck. It represents expression of your feelings, your ability to tell your truth, to convey what you mean using speech, and to trust that those hearing you want to hear what you express. To open this chakra, you can sing. You can say what you mean.

6. The sixth chakra or third eye chakra is also known as the Ajna chakra in Sanskrit. The color is indigo, and the seed mantra is "om." The note is A. The corresponding physical features are the pituitary gland, brain, left eye, the nose, ears and the nervous system. The symbol is a descending triangle within a circle, that is, the reverse of the fifth chakra (where the circle is depicted within the triangle). Here the circle is outside and around the triangle. This chakra is all about your intuition, intelligence, and psychic ability. You can write down or work with your dreams to develop your sixth chakra.

7. The seventh chakra or crown chakra on top of the head is called the Sahasrara chakra, and its symbol is the thousand-petaled lotus. Different teachings call this one by different colors: some say violet, others white, others gold. It corresponds to the pineal gland. This chakra is all about spiritual connection. Meditation and prayer keep the seventh chakra balanced and clear. The musical note is B. Its seed mantra is "om" recited silently.

The Hara

Hara is a term that originated in the medical system of Japan, and there it essentially means the soft belly, what in western medicine we would call the abdomen.

In Japanese medicine, this understanding of the hara is used as an area that reflects the health of all the organs—that is, their physical and energetic state of health as well as their relationships with each other. In Chinese medicine, the soft belly of hara, along with the pulses, is a primary method of diagnosis.

Jackson Morisawa, the Kyudo instructor at Chozen-ji in Hawaii, who lived to age ninety-two wrote:

> "Hara is the seat of Life, the center of intrinsic energy. It is also referred to as a state of mind in the development of one's character. One who controls the hara is not likely to lose his balance or composure. Who has hara

does not consume himself or spend himself completely. He learns to anchor himself in the hara, and can shake off disturbances of the body and mind and alternately release himself from the ego and return to the deeper power of the "original being." The will is silent, the heart is quiet; and one accomplishes his work naturally without effort."[24]

In the West, many mind-body modalities focus attention on the hara— including Alexander Technique, osteopathy, Feldenkrais, Shiatsu and massage. Brennan Healing Science also focuses attention on the hara, and Barbara Brennan considers the hara to be all about intention.

One way you can work with your hara is by standing with your feet about shoulder width apart, toes turned out slightly. Put your fingertips a few fingers below your belly button, and sense into the center of your body straight back from your fingers. Once you feel that spot in the center of your body, now sense that there is a pipeline that descends from that spot, through the center of your pelvis, down through your perineum, between your legs, down to the floor, down to the earth under the building you're in, and then all the way down, deep into the center of the earth. Allow yourself to root yourself there. At the same time, feel like your legs are like tree trunks. Let your "roots" grow down through your feet, all the way down to the ground under the building you're now standing in, down all the way, like we just traveled with the central pipeline, down each leg, to the center of the earth. Feel the support of your two legs, and the center pipeline, all the way up your hara. Now allow that hara line to extend upward from the point straight back from your fingertips in the center of your body. Allow that line to extend up as a pipeline in the center of your body, all the way up through your upper chest, through your throat, through your head, out the top of your head and above your head, about three and half feet (a little more than a meter) above your head. When you feel that connection, set your intention there, and feel yourself rooted into the earth, and, at the same time, extending up to the cosmos above. You may wish to say your intention out loud, or just feel it energetically in your pipeline as clearly and strongly as you can. Notice if your line feels strong, and what diameter it is. If you perceive that it's strong and thick—great! If it wavers or feels weak, bring your conscious awareness to your hara line, and see if you can envision and sense, using all your senses, your column grow thicker in diameter and stronger, more vital. If it is shaky, or your line is thin, you can use that awareness to ask, "Is this really my intention, and I'm just anxious or not trusting this is what I intend? Or does my intention not fit what I would really prefer?" This can be a jumping off point into further curious exploration.

Your Inner Light

So far, we have looked at the chakra system, which is all about you on the level of your personality, what we called the map of psycho-spiritual development. We've considered the hara, what some, like Brennan and Morisawa, consider the dimension of intention. There is another area of experience to consider, and that is what some in the West call your "essence," what here we'll call your own inner light, that is, who you are beyond the concerns of your personality, and all that you long for. Philosophers dating back to Aristotle and Plato, to more recently, Jean-Paul Sartre and Karl Marx have all written about essence.

At the level of essence, you are beyond the constraints of being in a human body or in any physical body at all. You may experience yourself as one with everyone and everything. Some people call this dimension the Soul. It may sound esoteric, but once you experience it, it becomes a palpable reality. You can perceive your inner light by feeling and seeing your entire body fill with light. To get there, you can use the Self-Tracking tool that we learned in the Assessment. First, go inside your body, and then fill your body with your own unique light. This light doesn't come from anywhere or anyone else; it is intrinsic to you. Each person's is unique.

As you do the Self-Tracking, and fill your whole body with your own light, now let it expand, so it is larger than your body. Let it shine more brightly; get bigger, so your light fills up all your chakras, your hara, and the energy field around your body. At the same time, let your light also, simultaneously, get smaller, so your own unique inner light fills up each of your cells. Now sense yourself as if you are a living pole of light, and let your light extend all around your body, 365 degrees around you, above, and below you. Now let your inner light expand further, so it fills the room you're in, then larger, so it fills the building you occupy. Let it get bigger—as big as your neighborhood, your city, your country. Expand further; get even bigger—as big as the earth. From here, it's easy to perceive what everyone you know and love is doing right at that moment. You can sense each of them wherever they happen to be, all over the globe. Now allow yourself to extend more, so you're bigger still. Go beyond the concerns of you in this body, in this lifetime. Go bigger still, beyond the concerns of being alive in a physical body at all. Keep going. Go all the way out to the edges of space, and you are like a lighthouse, beaming your unique inner light in all directions.

From this vantage point, it is easy to experience oneness. The concerns of the day, the worries that bother you on the level of personality, these fall away—and you are like a star, beaming your own inner light.

> *O to realize space!*
> *The plenteousness of all, that there are no bounds,*
> *To emerge and be of the sky, of the sun and moon and flying*
> *   clouds, as one with them.*

> - Walt Whitman, "A Song of Joys"

Voicework

We're now going to move into working with the sounds your voice can make, and here, too, the practices are physical, but they slide into emotional work as well. There are a few ways to work with your voice that can help you develop deep self-contact:

1. Make any vowel sound (a, e, i, o and u) with your voice. Take a deep breath and exhale as you make any musical note and sing or tone that vowel sound. At the end of your breath, let your voice trail off as you exhale every last bit of air. Let your abdomen contract to really squeeze out all the air. Repeat that several times, sounding the same note and same vowel sound, and let your voice trail off as you run out of breath. Keep doing this with the same vowel sound until a sound at the end starts to transform into a character with a message or "story" that wants to come through your voice. Play with what pitch to use to make the vowel sound. Different "stories" or characters emerge from different notes as your voice trails off. This may sound like singing or groaning or growling. It may give way to words or remain just sounds. As always, there is no right or wrong way to do this practice. Everything is okay.

2. Deliberately make animal noises or "ugly" sounds (groan, pant, hiss screech, scream, yelp, imitate animals who make loud sounds). It can be freeing to not have to make "pleasant" sounds.

3. Resonate through your chakras and make the sound of each chakra, as we learned above.

4. Now we'll learn Polish theatre director Jerzy Grotowski's Voicework that he developed for use with his troupe of actors.

We mentioned Grotowski above in the context of the "two scores" in acting, which we adapted for our purposes to represent what you listen for when working with clients to foster discernment. We described how Grotowski was interested in training his actors to be as expressive as possible, using only their bodies—no microphones, no lights with gels, no masks, and certainly not any artificial-looking, imitative sets—instead, he was interested solely in the body, in what the body can do. He called this "poor theatre."

How and why is this relevant for you? When you limit yourself to only focusing on what your body can do, you will likely find that a whole, rich world opens to you, where you can be enlivened, someone who is moved. Much like listening to a highly structured piece of music, a Bach invention say, you start to notice the flowering within the form, how much there is to explore within any given practice, for example moving, or using your voice. The catchphrase, "The body doesn't lie," can reveal your true feelings through these practices. They are again ways to help you connect to your sense of your own interiority.

Grotowski's actor training was rigorous, perhaps the most physically demanding approach to dramatic training that exists. The result is the body becomes "expressive," as we said, which is the opposite of "trained." Grotowski was obsessed with that distinction. He went further, and called a trained, but inexpressive body, "tamed." A gymnast works hard to train. The training develops the gymnast's body in a form that is ideal or perfect, within the forms of gymnastics. To get specific: As a gymnast, you execute certain movements, you assume particular positions, you pose in specific ways. But that's it. You're not trained to respond live and in the moment. You're not trained to generate or find new forms. Here's how Grotowski says it:

"{Gymnastics, like bodybuilding} makes a body
heavy, strong, even agile, but without any line of living
impulses, those almost invisible impulses which make the

actor radiant, which make that he is always speaking —even without speaking—not because he wants to speak, but because he is always alive. Gymnastics does not liberate, it imprisons the body in a certain number of movements and perfected reactions. If only some movements are perfected, then all the others remain underdeveloped. The body is not freed. The body is tamed. There's a big difference."[25]

In the context of the Thriving Through Cancer Method, like Grotowski's mission with his actors, and unlike a gymnast, you want to be able to feel every emotion and every sensation, and you want to be able to respond freely, not in any set, pre-ordained way, but rather live and in the moment. You want to be a vibrating, responsive, alive being, because a person who is that vital is, well, that alive, literally—you can enjoy excellent quality of life when you are that enlivened. Every nuance of an experience has the potential to resonate with you.

Interestingly, as Grotowski studied how to develop the voice in the most expressive way possible for actors, he developed a method of Voicework where you learn to use your voice through the chakras. There is no need for a microphone when you do this. He studied shepherds, who would call to each other across great distances. He was curious: How did they make their voices sound so loud? He discovered that they used their chakras, they resonate sound through the chakras.

Remember when we discussed vibration above in the practice to Track Yourself and the Other at the same time? When you work with your own voice as a reverberating, vibrating instrument, this connects you to your interior sense of yourself quickly, easily, and palpably. I mean that literally. You can put your hands on your clothes or skin and actually feel your body vibrate there as the breath passes through the chakras. And remember how we talked about the flow of energy being health, and stagnation of energy being disease? This practice of Grotowski's Voicework gets the energy to move right away.[26]

You can practice this in a group or on your own. When you practice in a group, you want to divide the group such that there are small groups of three to four people each, who each form a circle as they sit together on the floor. You want each group to have no more than four people so that they can position themselves with the tops of their heads very close, almost touching. If you're practicing by yourself, don't worry about that.

1. So now come to a kneeling position, and then put both your knees on the floor, so you are initially "standing" on your knees. Put your knees together and then sit back, so you're sitting with your buttocks on your heels. Now lean forward and put your elbows, and then your forearms down on the floor in front of you, your hands on the floor. Stick your butt up into the air. Relax your neck so your head is free; let it just hang down. Double check if you're tensing your neck, and if so, relax it so your head and neck are not exerting any effort to keep your head up. If you're doing this alone, you're all set. If you're practicing in a group, arrange yourselves in the circle we mentioned so your heads are nearly touching, but not quite. (By having your heads this close, you can perceive the group's resonance through your seventh chakra.)

2. We're going to make sounds—vowel sounds from particular chakras. The aim is to start to feel your chakras from the inside out—again we're developing our proprioceptive sense—how does this feel from the inside? We're not worried at all about how we look or how this sounds. We're going for the awareness from the inside of resonance.

3. So there's a trick for how to feel that resonance: you pump your belly in forcefully on every exhale, like bellows: When you want to inhale, you just relax your belly and the air naturally flows in. But when you exhale, you forcefully contract your belly button towards your back like a pump, to exhale the air. Try that now a few times.

4. So the chakra we're first going to sound from the first time we do this is your second chakra. As we discussed above, chakra means "wheel" in Sanskrit, and the wheels of our chakras are always turning. As we described above, the direction the chakras are turning is either taking in and metabolizing energy from the world around us, or losing energy. When each chakra turns clockwise, it means you're taking in energy there; counterclockwise means your field is losing energy there. When there is no movement, and the chakra is still, that means the energy is stagnant. Barbara Brennan teaches that the right hand rule of physics applies to chakras. To demonstrate this for yourself, you can use your right hand, and gently place your right thumb into each chakra. (Here's how it works: Barbara Brennan teaches that every chakra has a front aspect and a rear aspect. When you use your right hand both in front and back, you see that the chakras turn in opposite directions, when looked at from the outside.) Try this for yourself now: Extend your right hand in front of you. Raise your right thumb. Now place your thumb into one of

your chakras, say, the third one, which is right where your ribs separate. (You can refer to the descriptions under each chakra, above, to learn where each chakra is located on your body.) Notice with the thumb of your right hand in the chakra, the other four fingers of that hand can only turn in one direction. That direction is clockwise. That is, if you try to move your four other fingers in the opposite direction, your wrist gets in the way. Your hand can't rotate in that direction; it can't bend backwards. Again, you use your right hand in both the front and rear aspects of each chakra. By doing this, you see how the chakras turn in opposite directions (when you look at the front and rear aspect of each chakra from the perspective of standing outside the body looking at you). So the human body becomes a dynamo: clockwise is a different direction in the front aspect of the chakra as compared to the back aspect of that chakra; the same is true with top in relation to bottom (that is, the seventh and first chakras).

5. When we do the Voicework as Grotowski taught it to his actors, it helps you take in a lot of energy quickly. The vowel sound we'll use to get to know our second chakra is "Hoh!" And the position for this is the one I just described, with your weight resting on your elbows and knees, and your head hanging down between your arms, your butt in the air.

6. Now I'll summarize all the four chakras that we'll be doing this with for our exercise: As we said, the sound of the second chakra, as you forcefully exhale by pumping your belly, is "Hoh."

7. The next chakra we'll be sounding is the heart chakra, the fourth chakra, the one in your chest, right between your breasts. And for this chakra, the position is sitting up with your legs folded beneath you, knees apart, toes touching. You move from being on all fours, to sitting up that way. Here the sound of that resonator is "Hah," and it resonates from the center of your chest, your heart chakra. When we forcefully exhale, we say, "Hah." Again the second chakra pelvic vibratory sound is "Hoh," and the fourth chest vibratory sound is "Hah." The next one isn't exactly a chakra, but a powerful resonator, and that is in your sinuses. It tickles when you do it. The sound is "Heh." And for this resonator, you lean back and support yourself on your hands on the floor behind you so your chest points towards the ceiling. If that's uncomfortable, you can make fists with your hands and put your fists on the floor behind you as you lean back. This gives you extra length in your arms; you don't have to lean back as far. From that position, you resonate through your sinuses; it

sounds very nasal. The final resonator is the crown chakra, through the top of your head, and there the sound is "Hee." And you're again sitting up straight.

8. So to review: second chakra, "Ho!" fourth chakra "Hah!" Sinuses is "Heh!" and Crown is "Hee!"

9. And we forcefully exhale, make the sounds loud. So sit with your legs folded under you, in the circle. Lean forward on your elbows so your heads are close together, not touching but almost touching. Let your neck relax, and you can practice the breathing first. Pump your belly, by moving your belly button towards your back. Ex-hale! Ex-hale! Ex-hale! Ex-hale! In between each exhalation, let your belly relax, and then your lungs will naturally fill with air.

10. Okay, here we go. It's meant to be loud! If you do it all together, it makes a powerful sound. If you do it alone, it also works.

11. A good way to practice is to make each sound four times, and then move on to the next one. Then the third sound; then the fourth. Then start again. Do this several times. Remember the aim of this exercise is to start to feel your own voice resonating through your own chakras and resonators, to develop your internal, proprioceptive sense of yourself, from the inside out. As I said, you're not worrying about how you sound or look, but just going for the feeling from inside.

12. You can count three, two, one and begin: "Hoh, Hoh! Hoh! Hoh! Hah! Hah! Hah! Hah! Heh! Heh! Heh! Heh! Hee! Hee! Hee! Hee! And then repeat, several times.

13. Once you've completed that, if you're doing this alone, you might want to write some notes down. If you're doing this in a group, after you've done the exercise, come back together and share about it. What do you notice? How is that for you? Any emotions start to come up? Try speaking out loud. Do you notice a change in your voice? Is it deeper? You're learning how to let your voice drop from your head or throat down into resonating through your gut. Have you ever noticed how when you listen to certain speakers or leaders, their voice has a particular resonance? And how that resonance allows you to trust them? You believe they are speaking authentically. They sound that way because they are embodied—their voice is literally vibrating inside; we recognize that quality of embodiment as trustworthy.

So now we've covered the physical practices of the TTC Method, including eating for your bioterrain, movement from how it feels rather than how it looks, and we've referenced Sue Hitzmann's MELT method. We've learned about how to work with your chakras, your hara, your Inner Light, and you've learned several ways to explore your voice—letting characters emerge through you by sounding, making "ugly" sounds and imitating animals' sounds, singing the note of each chakra, and resonating through your chakras as taught by Grotowski.

Look at your worksheet now on "Putting Together Your Practices," and notice what your needs are physically. Do any of the practices draw you or feel like they might help you meet your physical needs? If so, write down which ones appeal to you on your Menu of Practices worksheet.

Next we'll move into the emotional practices.

CHAPTER FOURTEEN
EMOTIONAL PRACTICES

I remember the first time I looked at the spotless marble floor
> *of a giant hotel lobby*
>> *and understood that someone had waxed and polished*
it all night.

and that someone else had pushed his cart of cleaning supplies
> *down the long air-conditioned corridors*
>> *of the Sternberg Building across the street*

and emptied all two hundred and forty-three wastebaskets
> *stopping now and then to scrape up chewing gum*
>> *with a special flat-bladed tool*
>>> *he keeps in his back pocket.*

It tempered my enthusiasm for "The Collected Sonnets of Hugh
> *Pembley-Witherton"*
>> *and for Kurt von Heinzelman's "Epic of the Seekers for the Grail,"*

Chapter 5, "The Trial," in which he describes how the
> *"tall and fair-complexioned" knight, Gawain,*
>> *makes camp one night beside a windblown cemetery*

but cannot sleep for all the voices
>> *rising up from underground—*

Let him stay out there a hundred nights, the little wonder boy,
     with his thin blanket and his cold armor and his
               useless sword,

until he understands exactly how
     the glory of the protagonist is always paid for
               by a lot of secondary characters.

In the morning he will wake and gallop back to safety;
     he will hear his name embroidered into toasts and songs.

But now he knows there is a country he had not accounted for,
     and that country has its citizens:

the one-armed baker sweeping out his shop at 4 A.M.;

soldiers fitting every horse in Prague with diapers
               before the emperor's arrival;

and that woman in the nursing home,
     who has worked there for a thousand years,

taking away the bedpans,
     lifting up and wiping off the heroic buttocks of Odysseus.

- Tony Hoaglund, "The Hero's Journey"

Emotional Practices

When you're first diagnosed with any life-threatening illness, and at each new stage of the process, you'll likely go through a lot of feelings. One that may surprise you is suffering profound disappointment, as though your hopes, dreams, expectations, and plans for your life are changed quickly and utterly. Even if you know at the outset that what you have is curable, and you'll go on with your life afterwards and be fine, still, somehow, underneath, there's a sense of being humbled that seems inevitable: "Oh, so I don't have control over my life or body; I had heard about this. But now I see."

There's also a sense of joining the human race: "This just is the way it is. We live, and ultimately, we all die. We don't get to choose every aspect of our lives." And, "There's a story here; something has happened. Something is happening; it shapes me." Like Galileo Galilei stating, "And yet it moves," this much we know, about our human lives as well as the earth, if only we don't willfully refuse to ignore the evidence.

Before, if you had any idea that you are crafting your life, creating your life, being the hero of your own life, now you may experience a different, deeper call, and, like every call, one that inevitably leads you into trials you'd rather not confront, but find you must.

How you respond to this call, how you feel (or don't allow yourself to feel) your feelings, how you respond to being vulnerable and needing help, feeling physically awful, having feelings about dying—these experiences can forge you, if you choose to work with them that way. They certainly transform you.

So, personal bias: I believe if you let yourself work with your feelings and emotions, that's another way to get your energy moving again, another way to foster health. I don't believe working with your emotions is sufficient to cure cancer. But I do know that working with your feelings can help you feel better, weave loose ends in your relationships back together, and understand how you may have contributed to your disease process through self-abandonment or self-betrayal. Ultimately, you can use your emotions to galvanize your energy to choose how you want to live now. Living how you want to live, based on the wisdom you gain, might be the boon you can bring back from your journey.

That being said, now I want to say it differently, without the framework of mythmaking. It is not that we do these practices for self-improvement. It is not as though (even if we're sick), anything is wrong. There is nowhere to get to. Much as we humans love to make meaning and love to frame our experience, we love to use metaphors from battle ("I'm going to beat this!") or religion ("He's in a better place now; he's gone to be with God), or science ("The average five-year survival is x percent), the truth is, we're in the unknown. There are not always convenient truths. I believe that by being as present as possible, we can be as alive as possible. You can use the practices of working with your emotions to be as free as you are capable, even while in the unknown.

I believe it's for each person to decide if your illness reflects deeper issues. I strongly dislike when people suggest I "brought the cancer on myself," or it's my "karma," or anything that implies they can't stand the fact we can't seem to control it. (And yet sometimes I hate that I can't control it either.) We humans don't like to feel that cancer can just "happen," and while we have many clues, at this point we don't have a one-size-fits-all sense of causality for cancer, the way we do with many other diseases. Nowadays we talk about cancer not as one disease, but many diseases that are tied together only by uncontrolled cell growth.

In my case, I am curious about the fact that the cancer showed up some eighteen months after I first felt the profound disappointment with my modality and then left teaching at the healing school.

Turns out, I'm not the only one to be curious about this time frame from a traumatic event to the diagnosis of cancer. Back in the nineteen-sixties and seventies there was a husband and wife team that studied, theorized about, and developed a mind-body protocol for working with emotions and cancer. O. Carl Simonton, MD, a specialist in radiology and oncology, and his then-wife, Stephanie Matthews-Simonton, now a psychotherapist, together were pioneers in psycho-oncology. He died in 2009, and though they divorced before his death, she has gone on to found a different cancer treatment center.

Their research indicated that when lifestyle counseling was added to medical treatment for patients with advanced cancer, their survival time doubled and their quality of life improved. While their study design has been criticized, a 1989 study by Stanford and UC Berkeley researchers concluded that women who had advanced breast cancer who received emotional counseling lived twice as long as those who did not.[27] That study was seen to be independent evidence that the "whole-body approach" to treating cancer does make a difference.[28]

The Simontons' research, described in their book, Getting Well Again, seems to go in and out of fashion, but it is not considered to have any potential to harm patients.[29] Their theories interest me in that their clinical research at their oncology center suggested that many people who develop cancer do so around twelve to eighteen months after a traumatic event. Their profile of the "Type C personality,"—that is, someone who in childhood becomes wounded emotionally by some major disappointment, then grows up to find fulfillment by "putting all their eggs in one basket," or becomes devoted to one cause, only to re-experience disappointment again, and then cancer develops twelve to eighteen months later—that profile describes my experience. It also fits my mom's experience: She developed cancer and had her first mastectomy exactly—to the week—a year after my dad died. I've seen many, many women develop breast cancer after going through divorce or a breakup in their primary relationship. I realize this is just anecdotal evidence. Still, in my meaning-making state, I am curious about the notion that such profound disappointment seems to foster the growth of cancer that then gets diagnosed a year to eighteen months later. I suspect in time we may see confirmation about the emotional connection to the initial growth of cancer, much like we now know as demonstrated by the research we discussed above of Steve Cole, PhD, in which perceived social isolation "switches" gene expression "on" or "off" affecting the hormonal cascade and release of neuropeptides, which thus leads to earlier recurrence and wider metastases in women with ovarian cancer.

The Simontons noted another quality of people with the "Type C" personality: they typically are "very nice," "compliant" patients who take care of others to the exclusion of taking care of themselves.

Being "very nice" or "compliant"—in other words, more concerned with how everyone else is than how you're doing, even while you go through cancer— these are other ways of describing someone who is being outer-directed. If you know you need to learn to focus on yourself for your own health and well-being, how do you learn to do that, if you never learned it before? Based on the mind-body connection in psycho-oncology, here are some tools to work with your feelings that I find useful. You can experiment to see if they work for you, too.

Set Your Boundaries

Remember my story about family and friends around me saying things like, "Your situation is very dire!" or "You have to stay positive. Or death comes!" or "I wish you wouldn't dwell on it!" Every person going through cancer or any illness has a collection of remarks people have said, advice given, articles clipped and mailed or emailed, opinions shared forcefully, with a demand that the person receiving these must see the wisdom in what was sent and must therefore adopt whatever is the latest item they shared with you. When you read the online bulletin boards of patients sharing their experiences, this idea of setting boundaries—to preserve your peace of mind because everyone has an opinion about what you're going through— that's an area that garners a lot of posts, a lot of commiserating, and sometimes, some atrociously funny stories.

It's a learned skill to develop the strength to let in what you want to let in, and not take anything else on, but rather to set boundaries and refuse to caretake the people "sharing" what are actually emotional demands. It's not uncommon to lose relationships with family or friends over these "conversations."

That's the first of the emotional practices—to learn to not just be "compliant" or "nice" or a "caretaker" in the way the Simontons describe, but instead to set your boundaries however you want them.

Here are a few of my favorite stories of when and how I needed to practice boundary setting. See if these bring up your stories:

A woman I was friends with (but who lived in a different city, so our friendship was based solely on phone conversations and emails, plus a few conferences where we talked in person), on learning I was first diagnosed, shared how she, too, went through a "dark night of the soul." She said that, in her past, she suffered from acne. It got so bad that she found it affected her feelings about her appearance. She described how she was lying in bed one night, unable to sleep, and, "it got to be about ten p.m. And I called out to God, 'God, if you want me to suffer with acne, take me now!'" That was her dark night of the soul; she meant it literally, as in one night, her breakthrough coming at ten p.m. And she believed her feelings about having acne were equivalent to going through incurable cancer.

That was one of our last conversations, but in another one she shared the story of "Lizard Boy," asking if I had ever heard of him (I hadn't). She said, "Yeah, so Lizard Boy, I can't remember how exactly, but he lost his arm. And because he didn't believe in organized medicine, he had no beliefs about it. So, when his arm fell off, he just grew it back." She literally meant that if I didn't let my beliefs about medicine and healing and what constitutes cure get in my way, that I, too, could just regenerate and heal. She assumed that because I'm a healer, I agreed with her. (I did not.)

Similarly, someone I knew from healing school, who had dropped out after the second year, with whom I hadn't talked since (it had been some fourteen years), heard through the grapevine I had been going through cancer. He called me up, and proceeded to give many suggestions about diet, supplements, beliefs, esoteric rituals for healing. The pinnacle of his advice was, "Melanie, you're an energy healer! You were on the faculty of the healing school! Don't you think you can turn off your gene? If anyone would know that, it's you! Just turn it off!"

I can laugh about these conversations now. And certainly, if I knew there was a way to turn off the gene, I would. But at the time, I felt blindsided, as though in each case, I fell into some vortex of the other person's assumptions, that had nothing to do with checking if I agreed, or what I had tried already, or what my experience had been, or what I wanted. With all of these people, it felt like they couldn't handle my diagnosis, and so tried to demand (without admitting it consciously), that I caretake them. It took me several of these conversations, and other less preposterous ones, for me to learn to keep my boundaries, and not have the conversation at all, because I needed to keep my energy available for my own healing, not spend it on managing their feelings about my diagnosis.

So boundary setting is one of the Practices you may choose to use in your emotional response. This demand that you think or feel any particular way is frustrating, because ultimately that attempts to blame the patient—and not for just somehow causing the disease, but being "bad" somehow for not doing the one specific regimen that that person is certain will cure you. Of course, no one can make you feel anything if you don't let them, in other words, their "hook," needs to find the soft flesh of your vulnerability, and it can't if you don't bite the hook. Yet when you're already undergoing a lot, and you want to be in relationship with friends and family, it's easy in moments of vulnerability to let the hook wound you.

Become the Steward of Your State

From all I've said so far, you can tell that I believe that it's useful to feel whatever you genuinely feel. I've spent years championing that—that it's healthy to be authentic. I'm committed to that; I live that way.

Yet I want to add a caveat: If you want to, you may wish to experiment with "managing your state," not in the sense of faking how you feel, and certainly not in the sense of these friends who couldn't deal with feeling powerless, and so had agendas for me, but rather in the sense of assessing your true needs, and then consciously going about getting your needs met.

We mentioned Dr. Steve Cole's research about how perceived social isolation and loneliness affect how soon a woman recurs and how widely she metastasizes. I asked him, if we know that the key here is *perceived* isolation, that is, she feels alone going through ovarian cancer even if everyone around her loves her and wants her to survive, are we at the stage of prescribing "get some new friends," since we now know that upset, feelings of hopelessness and helplessness affect the release of neuropeptides and hormones? His answer surprised me. He said we know that perception of loneliness affects the blood chemistry for eighty days, much longer than just the day when you feel that way.[30] So, he says, "Plan your day accordingly!"

In my case, first I felt lonely because of my disillusionment with my modality. Then when we moved to Los Angeles, I felt lonely because we lived in a suburb so far away from friends that I rarely saw them. Yet I came to feel that, while unlike what my colleague suggested of just "turn off [my] gene," what I could do is do my best to be the steward of my own state. In other words, I could decide how to feel, at least sometimes.

So consider your own situation: If you know that the mood you're in affects your blood chemistry for eighty days, what state do you want to be in? What do you need to do to give yourself the best possible chances of keeping your blood chemistry on as even a keel as possible? Do you need more time with friends? Do you need to shield yourself from other people's projections, like those conversations I just described?

If You're the Doctor or Nurse or Caregiver

So far, we've discussed the framework for the emotional practices of the TTC Method if you're the patient. But what if you're the nurse, physician or therapist? How do you stay open emotionally, but not bite the hook of other people's assumptions, in order to caretake them? What boundaries can you set as a practitioner and how do you set them? As a physician, nurse, therapist, healer, and the like, how do you get your emotional needs met?

When I interviewed Dr. Asher at Cedars-Sinai (the doctor we mentioned who runs the post-cancer rehabilitation exercise program there, who examined me for lymphedema, and who co-founded and runs the Growing Resiliency and Courage with Cancer program), we talked about how the GRACE program works for patients with advanced disease. But we also discussed it from the point of view of the doctors. He said, The GRACE program was the last one that he co-developed "because we don't think about existential issues; that's hard for us physicians." He said,

"We typically have a busy clinic day. We worry about prescribing drugs, chemo, tumor markers. There's very little time to talk about what may be the most important stuff. What does this mean to you? How are we dealing with the fear? Gratitude? There's no time for that in a typical clinical day. When you have two hours to sit in a room with a group of people and say, 'We're going to talk about this entirely different dimension,' it's therapeutic for both ends. Doctors, as we all know, face burnout. A major reason is lack of time, the lack of when you don't acknowledge as a clinician the losses you experience, the sadness, the spiritual domain that is inevitable. If you keep going through the treadmill, it leads to cynicism or burnout."

Here we are again touching on the feeling of powerlessness, this time for the physician. Dr. Asher discussed how important it is emotionally as you go through cancer to feel powerful, but how cancer makes that not always possible. Instead, you can choose how you feel. Dr. Asher's program addresses this. He says,

"With GRACE, we saw a gap. For sick patients with metastatic disease, there was no systematic way to provide some strategies for people facing life-threatening illness. There's the gap, and the need. One person, one doctor, one patient, can't do everything. Bringing together people had already been done. Working on having a sense of purpose in your life, that had already been done. We aimed to package it all together and give a safe place to process all that arises."

He went on,

"It's so humbling to see, for example, a thirty-nine-year-old woman going through advanced cervical cancer, to see the amazing resiliency people can crystallize and bring forth. As a physician, I could never fully bring that out in a patient. But people in a group are healing themselves and each other through these six weeks in the GRACE program."

I asked if that support had any effect on the actual disease. He answered that he had "no idea if it [the program] has any effect on tumor markers. In other people's programs, higher progression rates are when people feel chronically lonely. That's been pretty well established," he said. "But," he continued,

> "I will say that when you bring eight or nine individuals together who are going through cancer, everyone's head nods. They understand each other. At the very least, we're hoping to share these strategies. If it makes any kind of impact on a tumor marker, we're not advertising it because it's not appropriate to give that kind of preliminary hope. But they can empathize with each other. They've walked in the shoes of another person. The program isn't intended to be a support group, though people are supporting each other. It's not a clique for five people. It has a beginning, middle and an end; it's a set curriculum."

In the program, they read Viktor Frankl's *Man's Search for Meaning,* and Naomi Remen's *My Grandfather's Blessings*, and *Kitchen Table Wisdom.* Dr. Asher says that they read and process one story each week.

Make a Structure to Feel Your Emotions

When you're the patient or the caregiver, one of the ways to work with your feelings is to make a structure—as Dr. Asher has done in his GRACE program—to feel what you feel and express it. You can start by working with your feelings alone through journaling, or Free Writing. But ideally, you also want to work with your feelings with another or a group (a therapist, a healer, a program or support group), because it's hard to do this deep healing work all by oneself. It's very human to need contact to work on our "stuff." We humans are social animals; we need each other. So having a structure (like the therapeutic hour or a six-week program) allows your feelings a safe frame in which they can flow.

Then, it's equally important to consciously change focus, so you don't spend all your time mired in feelings and become paralyzed, unable to live and instead "miss" your life. Dr. Barstis described this well at one of our first appointments. He said, "When you're [the patient, is] scared, you [the doctor] can't say to the patient, 'just don't worry,' but at the same time, you want to say to the patient: 'Go on with your life. You don't want to miss your life. You can worry all you want, and the same amount of time will go by. But you don't want to spend so much time worrying that you miss your life.'"

Kris Carr, author, filmmaker and cancer survivor, discusses her strategy of "three days of wallowing," in which when she would get worried or afraid, she would allow herself to "wallow," but for a maximum of three days. Then she would consciously change focus and get on with living her life.[31]

"Tie Me to the Mast"

Remember the story of Jason and the Argonauts? Remember the Sirens? The Sirens were beautiful creatures that were half woman, half bird. They sang beautiful songs that were said to lure sailors to their deaths. Jason was tempted by the Sirens' song, so he asked his sailors to "lash him to the mast"—that is, to tie him to the ship's mast so he couldn't be lured by the Sirens' tempting songs and so dash the ship on the rocks. That phrase "tie me to the mast" is shorthand James and I have adopted. You may wish to use it, too, or find your own. When I obsessively worry or feel afraid, or, in the past, when I would be in the throes of chemo sickness and couldn't remember that I'd ever feel better, James would remind me that, "This too shall pass." In other words, I should not get lured into thinking the situation is worse than it is or that it will never end. James is very good at this, and he's had a lot of practice, as I can get worried in a controlling way when I don't feel well physically. He typically says, if I'm in that state: "This isn't all of you; this isn't your only feeling. I know you're feeling (whatever I'm feeling right then—angry, sad, despairing, filled with doubt, worrying, afraid, any of the physical symptoms that so affect mood, too, like feeling nauseous, breathless, dizzy, etcetera) very strongly. But you won't feel this way forever." If I'm really feeling the worst, he'll say, "You've just got to get through this. You will feel better. You're not dying right now. You know how to do this; you're strong. Remember how you feel when you feel better? You'll feel that way again." Another version is for James, or my mom, or friends to remind me: "Don't try to decide anything; don't try to work on anything. Just rest now." Or the shortest, "Just go to sleep. Tomorrow's another day."

Remember Times You Felt Worse and Play the Worst Case Scenario

Believe it or not, it also helps to consciously remember times when I have felt worse, because then I can say to myself, "I survived that, and went on to feel much better, to enjoy many more months when I didn't think I would. If I survived that, I can survive this."

Similarly, it also helps to consciously envision the "worst case scenario." This strategy drives my family and friends crazy, because they fear I'm getting mired in not staying "positive." But if I allow my mind to wander into fantasies of what would be the worst that could happen based on what I'm experiencing now? That helps me identify what I'm having feelings about. It helps me determine my need—Do I need information? Pain relief? To talk with someone who can advise me what to expect? Far from being "negative," this "incessant worry," and being a "control freak," helps me manage and cope by identifying what's wrong. Once I know that and address those needs, I naturally stop worrying or obsessing.

Free Writing

Free writing is a method of journaling in which you write in longhand for a set amount of time, fifteen minutes, say, during which period the only rule is that you keep your pen moving steadily. You write about any topic you choose; the only rule is that you don't stop writing. If you get stuck, and don't know what you want to say, you simply write a phrase like, "I don't know what to write," over and over again until the next thought or feeling arises, and you write that. Popularized by such writers as Peter Elbow, Natalie Goldberg, and Julia Cameron, Free Writing is done without thinking about spelling, grammar, punctuation, etcetera. The aim is to discover how you really feel about any given topic, and if you're using it as a writing tool, as those writers describe, so you know what you want to say. For our purposes, journaling in this way is the best process I know to get in touch with how you really feel about something. Your journal becomes your own private space. It is great to do in a dedicated notebook, the same one every time you work this practice, so you can compare how and what you're feeling now with the past. It's important to practice Free Writing in longhand rather than typing on a keyboard as this helps connect you to your subconscious and hence your feelings, whereas typing seems to keep you in your rational mind. For purposes of the TTC Method, you can work the practice of Free Writing in two ways:

1. Write about any subject you want, even if you don't know a topic as you begin. This is a little like using Free Writing like a journal.

2. Write about a specific topic. You can either do this once on that topic, where you write for fifteen minutes, for example. Or you can write on the same topic for fifteen minutes, then take a break and do something else, without reading what you just wrote. Then come back, perhaps fifteen minutes later, and again write on that same topic for fifteen minutes. Repeat the process until you've written on that topic four times, for fifteen minutes each. Then don't read what you've written and instead go do something else for at least twenty-four hours. Then come back and read it. You can highlight or circle anything that feels true or right, meaning you get a jolt of recognition that feels like, "Yes, that's what I meant."

3. This is an excellent tool to help you break through any self-judgment, self-censorship, defenses and fears. If you're afraid someone else might read what you wrote and you're worried that what you actually feel is unacceptable somehow, this is your private space where you can explore.

Here are some topics you might consider to work with your feelings. Feel free to adapt these and/or add your own:

1. Are you living how you want to be living? If not, how do you want to live?

2. Pain—physical, emotional, mental, or spiritual.

3. The loss of who you were.

4. The presumed potential loss of who you might become.

5. Your own dying process.

6. Your own death.

7. What happens for your spouse/partner/family/friends after you die?

8. What's your legacy?

9. Any relationships where you feel you have unfinished business: What is wrong? What would you like to do to resolve and heal that relationship?

10. Changes in your body.

11. Changes in your emotional, mental, or spiritual life.

12. How do you betray yourself? Do you want to make different choices now?

13. If this were your last year alive (or month, or any variation that is true to your experience), how would you live differently? How do you feel in your body considering this? What if you live that way now?

When I worked these practices, I was shocked at how I kept confusing self-expression and self-betrayal. I came to see that I couldn't always discern the difference between these two behaviors, though they are very different. What I mean is: When I was first diagnosed, as is so common in cancer patients, I obsessed over the cause. And I'm someone who already knew I was at high risk because of having the BRCA1 gene. My thinking rambled: "Was it environmental? Or dietary? Or toxic burden?" I exposed myself to carcinogens in all these various kinds of ways, and sometimes not purposely, but either purely out of ignorance or out of being so disembodied, I just didn't make the connection that a known carcinogen might affect me, in my cells. Sometimes I may have put myself at risk of cancer out of a sense of overwhelm. This is not to act like a victim. Or to blame myself. Yet, for example, in the years before I got sick, I kept getting my hair straightened using Brazilian Blowouts, the ingredients of which, when combined in the heat process used to straighten the hair, apparently turn into formaldehyde. (The product was then under intense scrutiny and was the subject of news reports about its alleged possibility of causing cancer. Somehow despite having the BRCA1 gene, I just didn't put two and two together—it never occurred to me it actually might cause cancer in my body.) Also, twice I did a homeopathic version of the hCG diet, once before our wedding in 2009 and again in 2011, the second time for about a month. The hcG diet, even if "homeopathic," meant I was essentially dosing myself with a hormone that, if I were pregnant, would tell my body not to reject or attack the fetus as "foreign" or "other" and instead let the fetus grow to term. Might it be possible that that hormone communicated to my body that if my immune system detected cancer cells growing, it should similarly not recognize them as foreign? So my body, my immune system, could not, would not, go after cancer cells as "other" and attack them?

I am very curious about what is self-betrayal (the two examples of not accepting my: 1. curly hair—so straightening it using a product that essentially created the known carcinogen of formaldehyde, or 2. my slightly chubby state, and so dieting for the first time in my life before our wedding)? And what is just random, arbitrary, the intersection of all these environmental factors with the BRCA1 gene, that essentially tells my body not to suppress any tumor that might be starting, but instead to allow a cancer to proceed with growth: in a nutshell, to "make more cells"?

Add to this that the histology, that is, the cell type of the kind of cancer I had was transitional cell carcinoma. Usually that means bladder cancer, and the people who get it tend to be males who tend to work with leather dyes or chemicals all day. Some people who get transitional cell carcinoma are smokers. I've never smoked. According to Dr. Friedman, it's "weird" to get the unusual cell type in the fallopian tube cancer I had.

And how much of the cause was me being perimenopausal, when the natural balance of estrogen and progesterone goes through a shift? In my case, as in the cases of so many other women, I was likely estrogen-dominant, and the tumor was strongly estrogen-receptor positive. But I didn't know any of that in time to take actions to prevent it, and I don't know what, if any, actions I could have taken that would have been efficacious.

Live Your Tempo

Another way you can work with your feelings is to honor your own tempo in life. You can ask if you're spending time the way that best suits you. This self-acceptance is healing. In my body, it feels like such a relief: James and I laugh about this. He's fast at everything—he can shower and shave in ten minutes, he writes copy like he speaks, in one torrent. We have a joke that he can put up a website in the time it takes me to shower and put my makeup on. I do everything slowly. My natural tempo is slow. He's quick, but unable to focus on details. I'm slow and detail focused, but everything takes me longer. He gets a lot done; I get it done right. Usually we're a great team. But as I began to work with this practice of following my own rhythm, my body relaxed; it felt like I was sloughing off a habitual way of holding myself physically, specifically the way I held my muscles against my skeleton, with a lot of tension. I've come to recognize that for me, that tightness of muscle contraction is shame—I've always been embarrassed for how I do things. I've always apologized just for being me. As I began to notice that I often felt mortified just for being the person I am, and as I began to challenge that, I had all kinds of memories of judging myself and driving myself relentlessly, from early childhood on. This was my kinesthetic reality, my lived experience. As I became aware of that unspoken belief, and began to work with my emotions around it (why was I ashamed for being myself?) my body began to relax. I'm curious what effect that has on the cellular level.

So for you—in what ways do you judge or hate or shame yourself? Where did that idea originate? In what relationship? Usually it's in our families of birth, and often it's how we relate to our parents. Can you remember where you got the mistaken idea you had to be different in any way from how you naturally are? What might it feel like emotionally to say, "You know what? This is part of how I am; it's probably not going to change. So I'm not going to exert any more pressure on myself to alter this." What happens inside even as you read those words?

Now we've considered several practices to work with your emotions, including:

Set Your Boundaries;
Become the Steward of Your State;
Meet Your Needs Even if You're the Doctor;
Make a Structure to Feel Your Emotions;
"Tie Me to the Mast";
Remember Times You Felt Worse;
Play the Worst Case Scenario;
Free Writing; and
Live Your Tempo.

As with the physical practices, note which emotional practices draw you now on your Menu of Practices worksheet.

Next we'll move into the mental practices.

CHAPTER FIFTEEN
MENTAL PRACTICES

All the new thinking is about loss.
In this it resembles all the old thinking.
The idea, for example, that each particular erases
the luminous clarity of a general idea. That the clown-
faced woodpecker probing the dead sculpted trunk
of that black birch is, by his presence,
some tragic falling off from a first world
of undivided light. Or the other notion that,
because there is in this world no one thing
to which the bramble of blackberry corresponds,
a word is elegy to what it signifies.
We talked about it late last night and in the voice
of my friend, there was a thin wire of grief, a tone
almost querulous. After a while I understood that,
talking this way, everything dissolves: justice,
pine, hair, woman, you and I. There was a woman
I made love to and I remembered how, holding
her small shoulders in my hands sometimes,
I felt a violent wonder at her presence
like a thirst for salt, for my childhood river
with its island willows, silly music from the pleasure boat,
muddy places where we caught the little orange-silver fish
called pumpkinseed. It hardly had to do with her.
Longing, we say, because desire is full
of endless distances. I must have been the same to her.

But I remember so much, the way her hands dismantled bread,
the thing her father said that hurt her, what
she dreamed. There are moments when the body is as numinous
as words, days that are the good flesh continuing.
Such tenderness, those afternoons and evenings,
saying blackberry, blackberry, blackberry.

- Robert Hass, "Meditation at Lagunitas"

Mental Practices

As we move into framing the mental practices of the TTC Method, we broaden our perspective. We move away from looking at life-threatening illnesses only from the perspective of our individual human bodies (seen even down to the genetic or cellular level), or the physical or emotional issues that accompany that level of perspective, and now move into a more meta-perspective level—By that I mean we'll now connect to a more abstract, societal, global perspective. And what do we observe? As I write, headlines increasingly include reports about how we humans are changing life on the planet for every species.

We live in a time of massive change. Cancer is on the rise in the developing world and it is unclear if there is a causal relationship between the changes we observe and the increased rates of cancer in most countries. The earth is changing in that the effects of climate change are starting to affect daily life as we know it in, for example, massive, seemingly uncontainable forest fires, a greater number of super hurricanes and typhoons, algae blooms that turn bodies of water green and unsafe for both humans and aquatic life, visible seawater rise, and the start of regular flooding when the moon in full. We are being invited—constantly—to see the connection with every other living creature. The rate of change, if we absorb it, is shocking.

Since 1965, a hypothesis called the Gaia principle or Gaia theory has been put forth about the earth. Originally a result of chemist Dr. James Lovelock's work for NASA, concerned with detecting life on Mars, and later developed by Dr. Lynn Margulis, a microbiologist, it states, in a nutshell, that the earth is a complex, interacting system that can be thought of as a single organism.

While scientists argue about the theory, for our purposes, let's at least accept it as an analogy. From this perspective, the earth can be said to be a "body," and while the earth has no parents and cannot reproduce, still, at least metaphorically, it is useful to see the factors that interact and appear to have an effect on whether the planet remains habitable or not. From this perspective, we can see that the earth-as-body is going through changes, as we are in our individual bodies.

Many argue that we are in the early days of the sixth mass extinction: whereas the first five extinctions happened on earth due to cataclysms (whether we look at the volcanoes that may have caused the Great Dying, in which up to ninety percent of life on earth and in the water died, or the asteroid that ended the dinosaurs' dominance), this sixth extinction is being caused by humans. During the last several centuries, our use of energy, our building of larger cities, using land for logging or food, our growth overall has changed the climate for other species such that they are going extinct at a rate faster than in the past. Called the "Anthropocene defaunation" in scientific papers, we are seeing our human impact on biodiversity: more species are going extinct and those that survive are doing so with fewer and fewer numbers. Among vertebrates, it is estimated that three-hundred-twenty-two species have gone extinct due to human life since 1500, and among invertebrates, sixty-seven percent of monitored populations show a forty-five percent decline. Researchers think that such animal life declines will cascade into ecosystem decline and affect human well-being.[32]

When I first read those studies, the year 1500 sounded like a long time ago, and the phrase "affect human well-being," sounded manageable, like something we could learn to work around. But the latest research suggests global wildlife populations have fallen fifty-eight percent since 1970.[33] This same study suggests that by 2020 (a mere four years from today), that decline could reach two-thirds of vertebrates. The causes are said to be human activity, including pollution, climate change, and loss of habitat. Another study states that the earth is losing mammal species at twenty to one hundred times the rate of the past. Extinctions are happening so quickly that, within two hundred and fifty years, they could rival the event that killed the dinosaurs.[32]

We human mammals are also vertebrates. Do we think that the climate shifts and extinction of species we are seeing will affect all the classes of vertebrates, but not us? To come out of the abstract language for a moment, picture the familiar animals we take for granted, the birds, reptiles, amphibians, fishes, and other mammals—do we think that two-thirds of them will disappear soon, but not us? I realize my tone sounds both incredulous and blaming. Yet I can see that that possibility is similar to the way I just didn't seem to even notice or consider that if I used carcinogenic "beauty treatments," that they would affect me in my body, my cells—and this despite the fact that I knew I was at high risk. How could I be so asleep? The evidence suggests we are all entranced and unconscious about how these global changes affect us, even as we recognize that we are causing these same changes and we are starting to see evidence of them in our daily lives in the storms, algae blooms, seawater rise, and forest fires that we mentioned.

And I do mean to sound alarmist here. When I first began work on this chapter, I had a sense that in my lifetime we had all been subject to these sad environmental disasters, moments we knew about in this generation. That's only part of the story, however. There's a larger arc that is now becoming apparent.

Growing up there had been a handful of environmental disasters that affected my opinions, and gave me both a quiet rage (I was a teenager whose dad was dying of cancer; it was easy to project outward my sense of impending loss), and an existential feeling of insecurity, as though I didn't trust that it's safe to be alive in a human body on this planet.

I could tick these events off on my fingers: Starting with my thumb was the discovery as a teenager that carbon tetrachloride had been spilled into the Ohio River, where our drinking water came from in Cincinnati. It was not reported until after the slick had moved past us, so we all drank it unknowingly.[35] Next, I could count on my index finger Three Mile Island, the meltdown of the nuclear reactor in Pennsylvania which has been observed to have caused elevations in cancer rates in the surrounding area.[36]

On my third finger would be the Zimmer power station. When I was growing up, it was a delayed, endlessly under-construction and over-budget planned nuclear power plant that kept failing inspection for the safety of the welds on the pipes that would have carried radioactive water through the reactor. I recall articles about rates of leukemia and bone cancer being high in children around the plant, even though it hadn't yet started generating power. Photos of kids riding their Big Wheels in the pale dirt around the plant who then were diagnosed with cancer were the stuff of my nightmares. (Public opposition was so strong and the expense of bringing the plant to meet Federal safety requirements so high, that ultimately Zimmer never opened as a nuclear plant, and instead was converted to a coal plant.)[37]

On my fourth finger was the meltdown at Chernobyl,[38] with the accompanying food safety issues for crops grown in Europe, far but downwind from the plant, and ongoing health issues for people who lived in the vicinity. I remember that summer (1986) being told not to eat any tomatoes grown in Italy, quite a distance from what is now Ukraine.

Growing up in the nineteen-seventies, it seemed awful these events should happen, but it also seemed as though they just do. What I did not realize was that earlier generations had had their horrors, obviously, but not to do with this postwar industrial development and our widespread adoption of the use of powerful chemicals in our daily lives when we don't know how they affect us hormonally, physically, genetically, and epigenetically.

Rachel Carson's *Silent Spring* created the awareness of the effects of pesticides on bird and human life; her work spawned the ecology movement. In the seventies, her ideas were beginning to affect the mainstream. It began to be fashionable then to take actions to "save the environment." While Carson's work brought awareness of ecology, she personally died of breast cancer.

Now, in the twenty-first century, we see the arc of our chemical and more globally industrializing era more clearly, and it seems that no longer are we apathetic about the environmental disasters we cause, but the scale of the changes needed are no longer so easy to implement, the effects are more obviously rampant, and the changes needed seem more urgent, less a matter of chic convenience. For example, consider the water crisis in Flint, Michigan, in which an entire city's population was exposed to lead-contaminated drinking water for a couple of years. This contamination was a direct result of the city switching water sources, and not applying corrosion inhibitors to pipes, such that lead leached into the water supply. This was avoidable. But it was not prevented, and was denied by government officials for two years.[39]

Potentially affecting many more people, that is, all human beings alive, consider the issue of potential death and extinction of honeybees. Bees are needed to pollinate the fruits and vegetables we humans eat every day. Without them, crops cannot grow. Bees have been dying at alarming rates, with for example, up to seventy percent of bees in Iowa dying since 2006, and the honey production in California decreased by fifty percent in recent years.[40] With some saying the issue is not as bad as it seems—we know the causes now, we can address these, and bee colonies reproduce rapidly[41]—bees remain vulnerable, and our seemingly it's-just-human-nature ethos to choose short term "fixes" rather than long-term common-sense policies has not been solved.

So in the midst of this awareness, how do we respond? One way is to become politically active, to address these global needs from societal, governmental policy and regulatory frameworks. Another, perhaps related way, is to utilize technology to share resources, brainstorm ideas, and share best-practices strategies. I see the decomposing quality of healthcare in the US as being a parallel and related breakdown of the environmental and societal changes that are beginning to be ubiquitous. During the industrial era, in the not so distant past , the specialization of medicine, and even considering the body as a series of "systems" made sense: The field of allopathic medicine became more than one person could learn, so, because the paradigm of industry seemed so right, that led to specialization. Just like a factory worker knew one task and performed it repetitively and well, with an economy of gesture and focus, so, too, did medicine become structured with each doctor centered on becoming highly skilled in one area.

Yet now in the West, we are living in a post-industrial age. One person cannot possibly memorize everything, yet nearly everything one could need to learn is available online. From people with rare diseases finding each other and sharing information, to every symptom and what it could possibly mean (along with suggestions of what to do about it), being readily available, technology facilitates a new style of learning, practicing healthcare, and structuring all fields of endeavor. Potentially more holistic, it is also less about competition. Already the benevolent entrepreneurs of our age (Mark Zuckerberg, Bill Gates, Oprah Winfrey) spend their wealth on collaborative models of medical research and education—this is spawning the development of new drugs faster, even as no single team can claim solitary achievement of victory. Books about cancer are no longer just books; they invite a community of readers to share information and strategies. See for example, Kelly A. Turner's *Radical Remission, Surviving Cancer Against All Odds.*[42]

So we are in the death-throes, I believe, of the short-lived but suffering-inducing practice of medicine with such an emphasis on profit at the expense of patient care. It doesn't work for anyone—patients, doctors, nurses, or employers who must provide coverage.

So now narrowing this wider scope back to the personal, and what we can do to solve all this mentally, what is called for? How can you use your smarts to help you? What practices can you implement that can give you excellent quality of life?

Putting Together Your Team

We talked already about how you can recognize that physicians are human beings who have different personalities. Dr. Asher reminded us that you can't expect to make your physician someone they're not. He gives the example of choosing a surgeon: "You may not want to go to him for all the 'fuzzy stuff' but if he's a great surgeon, who cares? You can still find your integrative care from other practitioners," he said.

So how do you find your team?

I asked Dr. Friedman how he works (And, by the way, he's a great gynecologic oncology surgeon, who's also good at the 'fuzzy stuff'—he's the physician I described above who is known both for choosing his specialty because he thought, "I can do this better," and for delicately removing every bit of carcinomatosis, those little "rice-Krispies"-like tumors that tend to occur everywhere in a woman's pelvis with ovarian cancer. If you leave even one, they quickly grow back. That's part of what makes ovarian cancer most often a fatal disease.) As a healer, I'm interested in a warm connection between doctor and patients, and I'm interested in what, specifically, a surgeon feels—literally. How does he work? What does he perceive?

Since I personally experienced the trust Dr. Friedman instills in everyone, I became even more curious. When I was in the hospital, before and after the operation with him, so many nurses whispered, "I go to Dr. Friedman. I bring my daughter to Friedman." He described his popularity this way:

> "They perceive that I know what I'm doing and actually care about them. Which I do, obviously. But the whole issue of what I see and feel in surgery—a lot of this is what you feel in your fingers. I feel it underneath the tissue covering. You need to be able to define planes between tumors not with your eyes, but your fingers, because you can't see those areas."

I asked what that feels like.

> "It feels harder," he said. It doesn't feel like normal tissue. It feels stiffer. Lots of times for ovarian cancer, you'll see bumps all over things. You're stripping the diaphragm because you feel little bumps on that or on the peritoneum, like sand or golf balls, flat-bottomed golf balls, like a hemisphere."

He also answered,

> "How to choose a surgeon? You want someone who does specialize in gynecologic oncology if that's the kind of cancer, but who has a whole range of abilities. I know the people I'd let operate on me. It's hard to pick the really good ones and the ones who are not so good. Those of us in private practice" [as opposed to academia] "don't get students. Those of us in private practice often end up doing way more surgeries. I do fifteen a week; they do two to three a week. I've seen some really good people in private practice. And it's really highly variable."

Dr. Friedman, as you can tell, obviously impressed me.

At the same time, I chose for my hematologist-oncologist, that is, the doctor who would follow me and treat me with chemo, Dr. John Barstis. In my case, because of my genetic status, and knowing taxane drugs don't always work so well in people with the BRCA mutations, he bumped up in the queue the Doxil (called Caelyx in the European Union)—in other words, we used it for my first recurrence, when that's unusual: As I mentioned above, he had a creative strategy to keep me alive and strong with my bone marrow able to recover, and my blood counts intact, so I could be alive and vital enough to take advantage of the PARP-inhibitor drugs he knew were coming down the pipeline.

The two doctors have distinct styles, and practice at different institutions. I found them via Chris Bledy's book, *Beating Ovarian Cancer*. I have a strong memory of reading her book in the middle of the night. When I realized she, too, lived in the Los Angeles area, and she had survived recurrence, I looked up her doctors' phone numbers, and the next morning made appointments with each. I changed my team, and I, too, am still alive.

So what qualities do you want? Someone who's brilliant? Someone with an excellent bedside manner? Someone who works with you to preserve and bolster your quality of life? Or perhaps someone less warm-hearted, but who will do everything humanly possible to keep you alive?

Medicine is changing. Remember my story of my prophylactic breast surgery and reconstruction that I described in the chapter on Remission and Prophylactic Surgery? I found Dr. Minas Chrysopoulo, a great human being, and a very skilled, delicate surgeon, through the FORCE (Facing Our Risk of Cancer Empowered) website. Contrast that with my appointment with a different potential surgeon, who spent probably two hours holding forth on the various surgical options (which I had already researched), none of which was relevant to my situation, since I hadn't had breast cancer. All of the choices made me feel if I let him operate on my body, I'd feel disfigured: He knew the standard procedures—he could take skin from my back or thighs to make me new breasts.

When I tried to tell him I had already researched these methods, and the options were not what I was looking for (requiring three surgeries, expanders, more major scars), he grew incredulous. I can still hear his voice and picture his face with white hair, his funky black clogs, as he said, "You found him from a website?!" when I described the new, better way of doing the surgery. Neither would he let me look at any pictures of results on any women's breasts he had operated on. Dr. Chrysopoulo has women so pleased with our results we volunteer to talk to each other, and post on online bulletin boards by the hundreds, describing how happy we are with the appearance and sensation we still have in our reconstructed breasts. Pictures of women who've gone through the various procedures are directly available (and anonymous) on the website. So medicine is changing, partly as a result of technology. You, as a patient, get to have many more choices than in the recent past. You get to choose what qualities you want in your team, what results you want (in my case, to look as natural as possible, to do so in one surgery, without expanders). It's worth researching and advocating for yourself.

Dr. Chrysopoulo loves social media as a tool for advocacy and spreading the word that the new surgical techniques can be done successfully. Here's what he said about it:

"Social media is a window into the future of medicine. People active on social media are twenty years ahead of the rest of the population in the ways they view healthcare, seek information, want justification for certain decisions. I love Twitter. There's no BS on Twitter. You can post a link with a scientific article, and discuss it with people halfway across the world. I hooked up with a guy two years behind me in med. school. We're all advocating for breast reconstruction in patients with the BRCA gene. It's great. Patients are being armed with questions to think about. There's no stumbling block. The question is, will their doctors listen. The practice here (in San Antonio, Texas) has changed since the time I came on board. I notice the level of education potential patients are already turning up with. There's the progressive physician type and the dinosaur. Hopefully, in ten years' time, there will be more use of social media for education and discussion."[43]

This story has a lovely postscript. After my successful breast surgery, I volunteered to talk with other patients. A few called, and one of them has become a friend. Facing the same genetic risk, it was very helpful to share tools and suggestions with each other. We met for coffee a few times in California, and immediately ran into the ladies' room at restaurants to compare results. We're both quite pleased.

When I interviewed Dr. Chrysopoulo for this book, he also addressed the changing field of medicine in terms of the problems in the current iteration of healthcare this way:

"I don't want my kids to go into medicine," he said. "For a massive number of people, it's disingenuous—that is, it's 'outcome based,' but only in terms of 'let's look at outcome in terms of physician performance.' All that would be great, except we're just not seeing that to be the case. The insurance companies are not looking at all outcomes, but rather outcomes that suit them to back up what they want to do. We see that in many facilities. Doctors aren't able to have an honest conversation. Most physicians are employed by other entities. There is a change of culture brought about not by generational shifts or succession planning. But there's a new generation of physicians coming out. They don't want to work hard, or fight these battles. They want to clock in, clock out, and go home. Their way is to make it more of a shift system. We see it repeatedly. We're disappointed by the lack of what appears to be physicians being domestic. The practice of medicine is being replaced by shifts. With ER physicians, it has to be a shift system; I'm not including all specialties in this. But when you have some of your sub-specialty colleagues. They complain when we call and say we tried to get in touch with the physician. The doctor didn't want to talk because he was not on call, but it was his patient. Medicine is changing. What we talked about before with social media and so on leads to personal customization, shared decision making, self-advocacy, all this revolution going on. Yet on main street, medicine is a shambles. There's a split. I don't know where it's going to go."

This is spoken by a man who's part of a small, highly skilled, highly specialized group practice, that has worked hard to establish agreements with every possible health insurance company in the US, so patients can come for this specialized surgery, and have it covered by insurance.

In the midst of this shifting dynamic within the field and structure of medicine today, here are some tools that you can use to work with your mental level to keep yourself clear, organized, and able to choose what you want as you go through treatment:

Medical Binder and Index

Start a medical binder to stay organized. Ideally this is actually a combination of a big accordion folder, along with a binder. Use the accordion file to store medical records, in chronological order from the earliest (on the bottom of the stack), to the most recent on top. Always get copies of your medical records, or download them from your hospital's website. Your compilation of records should include everything: every blood test, surgical report, pathology report, every visit summary, every round of chemo including what you were given in its precise dose with what pre-meds and what anti-nausea meds in which doses, and every medication you have been prescribed in your treatment. If you've done radiation, note the total dose, and how many appointments you had. If possible to note the dose at each appointment, that's even better.

Also make an index of these records. I like to organize it as a table. The first column on the left is a number, with 1 being the most recent, and each progressive number being an item further in the past. The next column from the left is what the item is (e.g., specific tumor marker result, bloodwork, chemo orders, etcetera), the name of the doctor who ordered it, and where it was done. The third column is the date, again with the most recent on top and each lower row moving back in time. Finally, the fourth column is a summary of the results.

If you want, you can buy those numbered tabs that fit into looseleaf notebooks, and use a looseleaf instead of the accordion file to keep your records. You can also use those files that lawyers use for exhibit files. With those, the metal holder goes through two holes in the top, and the numbered tabs get stacked progressively with the numbers showing down the right side of the file, separating each item. The numbers of each document correspond to the number in your Index. That way you can reference any document immediately by looking for its corresponding numbered tab in your roster.

But if you don't do choose to use the numbered tabs, just paper clip your records one by one and stack them up in reverse chronological order in your accordion file.

I also recommend scanning all your records, and keeping them sorted by each test name, blood test, etcetera, and date. This allows you to see on your computer all your results sorted by what type they are: for example, all your tumor marker blood test results all in one place, all the pathology reports together, etcetera.

If you're in the US, and you have a lot of medical bills or claims coming in, you can file those, too, also in reverse chronological order, in another section of the accordion file. I didn't keep an index of those, because my various insurance companies in the US over the years had websites that displayed the claims organized chronologically.

You also want to keep a running list of your questions that you'll ask your doctors, and your doctors' responses. You can keep those in your binder, if you'd like. I kept those in my paper calendar (which is in a small looseleaf binder) on blank pages behind that month. At the end of the month, I'd pull out those questions, answers, and notes and file them. You'd be surprised how useful it is to have those notes sometimes years later when you can't remember details of medications or doses or other questions you had in the past that become relevant again.

It's helpful to both you and your physician to organize and write down all your questions ahead of each appointment. It's also helpful to go with someone to your appointments, so you can remember what was said. If one person is taking notes, and the other is listening, you'll usually end up with some version of what was actually said at the appointment. You can also record the conversation on your phone. When you're the patient, it's a lot to go through to organize your questions and then deal with any emotions that come up as you discuss how you're feeling with your doctor. You also want to include in your binder a running list of your symptoms and how they change as you go through treatment. It's worth keeping a list of all your changing at-home medications, too, and how you do on them, which side effects affect you.

Research

I have strong opinions about researching. Several times, I've started to look something up and have not been able to gather a full picture, so I've worried unnecessarily and made myself insane. I would love to say I've improved at this skill, but sometimes I still draw the wrong conclusions, or out of fear, when I'm in a hurry, interpret facts incorrectly. A classic, funny-but-not-funny example is from the first month after I was diagnosed. I had gone for a blood draw one afternoon before flying to Texas to get a second opinion at MD Anderson. This was maybe a week after the first surgery; I was still a newbie in the world of cancer, not feeling great physically, exhausted, and still in shock emotionally. As I sat at the airport en route to that appointment, the results arrived via a link in my inbox. When I logged in via my phone, I saw my blood showed elevated calcium. I began to research what that could possibly mean, and the news wasn't good: high calcium levels can mean cancer has metastasized to your bone. I got frantic. And then it was time to board the plane. Then time to shut off all electronic devices, and I tormented myself and James nonstop all through the flight, that evening, the next morning, the beginning of the appointment.

Finally, the next afternoon, after Dr. Pedro Ramirez at MD Anderson had examined me, James and I met with him and a panel of oncologists. Sitting in a circle in a nondescript conference room, they were a veritable round table of white coats, with years of experience and education between them, punctuated with James and me in our expressions of ignorance and fear about what lay ahead. When I began to ask questions, of course, I blurted out immediately, "Do I have bone mets?" The room of doctors in their white coats went silent. Dr. Ramirez cocked his head, furrowed his eyebrows, looked at me, chuckled, and said, "What? That's extremely unlikely." Then he asked, "Wait. You think 'cause your calcium was elevated in your blood work, you have bone mets? Had you just eaten lunch before the blood test?" The results were time-stamped 2:00 pm. I nodded yes. That's how I learned your calcium goes up when you eat. It was nothing to worry about. James turned to me with tears of relief in his eyes, and, in this formal medical meeting, blurted out, "You dork!"—our longtime term of endearment towards each other. Tears sprang to my eyes, too.

Over the years, many physicians and nurses have warned me to "Stay away from 'Dr. Google.'" I know why they say that. Obviously I'm not the only person who goes to the worst-case scenario when I get anxious. And in the next chapter, we'll explore how to research with discernment and not just to support you in your (inevitably) preexisting biases. I understand why before they get to know me, doctors would be concerned about my researching, but I disagree. If you can learn by reading reputable and scholarly articles, and have patience to work through the unfamiliar terminology, research can give you useful information to make decisions about your care and treatment. Not only scholarly websites and journal articles are helpful, however. Websites where people share their experience are also often useful. Often people share tools to cope with side effects. For example, it was through online bulletin boards that I learned that putting ice on your hands and feet and slurping ice in your mouth during Doxil infusions can help mitigate the blisters that can appear on your palms and soles in hand-foot syndrome and prevent the mouth sores (all common side-effects of Doxil). You can look at all these sites, and you need to practice discernment. We'll explore that in the next chapter.

Research can help make you powerful rather than powerless. When you read studies, learn of patients' experiences, understand various treatment regimens, you come to your appointments better equipped to choose what you want. Then you can treat your team as a resource, as fellow human beings who have experience working with people going through cancer. That's beneficial.

Then there's a time to stop researching. Under Emotional Practices, we talked about how Dr. Barstis tells his patients to go on with their lives and not get mired in worrying, because the same amount of time will go by either way, and you don't want to miss your life. He also talked about turning off your inquisitive mind and consciously choosing to change focus. He put it this way:

> "How to work with your state of mind? That's one of the hardest things for me with my patients. I'm always trying to get clues about how to help people get the most out of life. I know they're going to live a long time. But I know how it is. I can't stop thinking about a problem until I solve it. But that doesn't work. At a certain point, you need to give yourself time, shut your brain off, and do other things. That's the biggest challenge. They're going to live for a long time. Thirty years from now, when you're still alive, and all you did was think about your cancer, okay, what do we do about it? What we ought to be doing about life, few of us can. That's the practical aspect with my patients. I do my best to figure out their brains and understand what it is that's bothering them."

That's true service. What emotional intelligence: Someone who can figure out how you think so he can best help you—that's true personalized medicine. So why research? Because knowledge is power. Learning about what you're going through is one way to be proactive and decide what you prefer.

Chapter Sixteen
More Mental Practices

"You cannot find peace by avoiding life."

- Virginia Woolf

Be Proactive

This whole book is about being proactive, that is, actively doing what you can, what you choose, to have the life you want as much as possible, even in the face of life-threatening illness. A generation ago patients were not expected to be proactive. There was an unspoken assumption that one should "just trust the doctor. He's the expert." (And the reality was, that doctors in that generation were almost all men, and white.) Now, however, with the view of the patient-as-consumer being part of the Zeitgeist since at least the nineteen-eighties, there's a democratization of medical knowledge (just as there is with every kind of knowledge). When you are the patient, it's perfectly acceptable today to advocate for yourself, to ask questions, research, and do everything in your power to survive.

When you're the clinician, it's helpful to give guidelines to your patients that encourage them to be proactive. I loved when Dr. Barstis asked me at our third appointment, "Did you have a chance to think about whether you'd consider trying Doxil for chemo?" You can hear the empowering tone of his question, the assumption that we were partners in doing our best to try to help me survive as long as possible, and ultimately, he was offering me a choice of how I wanted to go about doing that. I hadn't known until that moment, though he had asked me to consider Doxil at the second appointment, after he had reviewed my case, that he really meant it—I had not emailed him between those appointments because I thought when he suggested I "think about using Doxil" that he meant it rhetorically. But as he asked me, I reported to him what I had learned that week from my research. I got to ask him all my questions and express my concerns about hand-foot syndrome, mouth sores, the then-newsworthy shortage of the medication, etcetera. He answered from his experience, and to me as the patient, that felt like together we designed the protocol for my treatment. I learned he preferred email to phone, when he wanted to hear from me between appointments, even if nothing was bothering me, to check in and see how I was doing. This was clear; I could do that. I felt seen and like I could trust him; I believed he cared about my well-being and we were on the same page. Setting the groundwork in these early appointments meant that as I'd have moments of fear going through the treatment, I trusted him and the system of communication we had put into place. This can go a long way towards relieving anxiety for a patient. (The opposite is all too common: you don't know when or how to reach out to the doctor. That's not empowering; it increases anxiety.)

If you're the clinician, you can hear how giving guidelines to your patients that encourage them to be proactive makes your work more interactive. I believe that can keep your busy practice meaningful (As opposed to feeling you're on some treadmill, forced to see patients as quickly as possible to meet your nearly-impossible-to-maintain contractual obligations to the health insurance companies.)

So, let's talk about what not being proactive looks like and the results. This is anecdotal, obviously, but see if you recognize any familiar (yet all too human) behaviors in these stories. We've all been there—maybe shy, maybe in denial, just wishing something would go away. That doesn't go well. This is not the time to doubt yourself, or to think everybody other than you is right about your experience or symptoms.

I had a friend who had cancer and has since died. She was someone I had known since high school, though now we lived in different cities and had lost touch. A mutual friend reconnected us, and since we were both going through gynecological cancers, it was easy to talk often and compare notes.

In our phone conversations, I was always struck by how passive she was being. She had ignored not feeling well for months. Then she had had a hysterectomy. She didn't know what kind of cancer she had; she had not attempted to find out. It's unclear to me, though I asked her, if the doctors knew—was it an unknown primary? Or did she just never read the pathology report? Bumps had appeared on her incision. She again waited months to get them checked out. Had she researched, she would've learned that incisions are common spots for recurrence. Her primary care doctor in her small town in New England thought they were "nothing," and she didn't question him or find a gynecologic oncologist and go for an appointment. (Research states clearly that survival in gynecological cancers is improved when the woman sees a doctor in that narrow specialty, gynecologic oncology.) She still didn't feel well, and now had fevers every afternoon, and sweats every night (classic signs of cancer). And she would insist, "Melanie, I don't know why you say it's so hard to survive recurrence." And "My husband tells me he won't let me go," and he was a doctor. This was striking to me—as though her husband was omnipotent and could simply will her to live, because he'd miss her if she died. Our approaches were so different. She died less than a year later.

If you're the practitioner, you need to respect what people want. If they don't want to know, it's important to honor their decision.

But I think often people don't know how to question, or they don't know they have the right to question. They don't know which questions to ask. Or they can't deal with the emotions that arise when they contemplate asking: "What if I'm sick? What if this is not nothing?" As a practitioner, you can help them. Ask your patient specific questions, "How are you feeling since your surgery? Any new symptoms?" Or, "You have bumps on your incision? Show me. Let's discuss. Hmm. I don't think those are anything, but let's find you a referral to a specialist." Or "You have a fever? How long has it been going on? What's your temperature? Is it every night, or were you sick and then it went away?" Or, "How are you feeling emotionally since the surgery? Anything you're worried about?" These are likely obvious questions to you if you're a practitioner. But what if, sensing the two scores we talked about in the Assessment, you perceive that the patient is deferring to your assumed authority—by not asking questions, not revealing much? This might show up in them being fidgety or not making much eye contact, or looking at their partner in the room, who presumably has heard the patient's worries. You can name what you notice: "I know I'm the doctor, and you're the patient, and maybe you think you're supposed to just trust me and follow along with what

I say. It's true you can trust me, and I notice you're being really quiet. I'd like to really hear how you're feeling, if you're willing to share it."

Usually, if you invite the client to share so directly, something will shift—either the patient will tell you something, or her body language or eye contact will shift. Then you can follow that, and ask more questions.

Patients, it goes without saying, but if you attempt to talk honestly with your doctor, and your physician can't meet you there, or dismisses your concerns, or in any way does not welcome your input, that's not a great doctor. You can switch; choose someone else. I had a doctor like that. It took me several appointments to decide to leave, but I knew when I'd come out of each appointments that I felt dismissed, like the doctor was numb and more concerned with fame and getting grants than monitoring me as I headed towards recurrence.

Here's another example, not cancer-related:

My "California Mom," my mother-in-law, Dee, had a red patch on her inner arm, under her skin near her inner elbow. It was spreading, moving up her arm. Within a few hours it was bigger and redder. She thought it was a skin issue. We were on vacation together. My father-in-law and James initially said, "Get some skin cream. Maybe it's dry skin." They were a little dismissive as we all wanted to go on a hike. The next morning it had spread further and was redder. It was making her skin look blotchy over more of her arm than the day before. I was concerned it was a staph infection, based on past experience. We were at brunch, everyone was brushing it off. I found I could not ignore it. My in-laws have a concierge arrangement with their primary care doctor. I insisted that we call him. Right there at the brunch table, we took pictures with her cell phone and emailed him the images. He immediately called back; he, too, was concerned it was a staph infection. That can turn deadly in a matter of days, and it was clearly worsening. I had looked up online a nearby pharmacy and their phone number. Right away he faxed a prescription for an antibiotic to the pharmacy and we picked up the pills right after brunch. She started with the first dose immediately. The next morning the redness was diminished and was now shrinking back to her inner elbow again. Had we waited, she would've grown sicker, and possibly died.

How did I know it might be staph? Unfortunately, from past experience: A friend of my parents' returned from a family trip, an African safari. He hadn't noticed that he had a cut or mosquito bite that got infected, that similarly spread through his bloodstream. By the time he returned to his midwestern hospital, and the doctors there didn't think to ask him whether he had been around mosquitoes or living in a tent recently, they didn't immediately think to look for a staph infection until it was too late. He died within days.

Because I had seen a picture of him on that trip and inappropriately blurted out, "Oh, look, his leg's swollen. You can clearly see the spot on his shin where the bite or cut happened, and his whole leg is swollen. How sad!" People were angry with me, but when I saw a similar redness on Dee's arm, I wouldn't let it drop. I immediately looked up images online of staph infection, and compared those to her arm. Convinced this was a real issue, I became controlling and tenacious; I could not just talk about pleasant things at brunch, until we called the family doctor.

So these are just a couple of examples. Being persistent, dogged even, is important. If something doesn't seem right, don't wait too long to see someone who can test or assess if there's cause for concern or not. This is another way of saying that ultimately, we each need to be responsible for our own health; we need to be the "captain of our own ship." Kris Carr discusses this in her book, *Crazy Sexy Cancer Tips*.[44] Regarding choosing your team, she describes it as you interviewing a potential CEO for the very important job of "Save My Ass Technologies, Inc." Regarding doing your research, she's all for it. We've drawn different conclusions. The natural regimen that worked for her didn't work for me. (I wish it had.) But she's all for advocating for yourself. She also discusses being willing to travel—and describes studies that show that those who are willing to travel more than a short distance, do better. Being willing to travel is another way of being proactive to save your life.

Travel for Better Care

I would add that not only is it worth traveling to a nearby city, but it's worth it to travel or even immigrate for better care. For example, the new PARP-inhibitor drugs (the amazing, new oral chemotherapy—pills, not infusions—that work by killing the "bad" cancer cells, but don't harm the "good," healthy cells), these are shown to be potentially highly effective in people who have the BRCA gene mutations. Yet as I mentioned at the beginning of the book, these are not covered by the health insurance I had in the US. The first one to be approved by the FDA, olaparib, costs $13,500 per month in the US. I got a letter from my insurance company in California at the end of 2014; they just wanted to let me know that any oral chemotherapy drugs that might get approved, would not be covered under my plan. And there was no other plan available that I could buy in my ZIP code as a self-employed person.

In the Netherlands, where we now live, that same medication, olaparib—should I need it in the future, is covered at one hundred percent. We did not know that when we decided to immigrate. This is not at all why we moved here. We expected I was almost done with treatment and would be back in remission. We did not know that drug would be covered, or even what health care was like here, except from hearing that our Dutch friends are satisfied with their care. We couldn't see doctors and learn this until we had immigrated and gotten health insurance. But the fact that the first PARP-inhibitor is covered, just seems like the right allocation of healthcare spending. Why would a health insurance company not want their patients to do well and go back into remission as quickly as possible? It's less expensive for them to have fewer patients who need treatment and more in remission, with patients paying our premiums but not using resources.

Medical tourism already exists for plastic surgery. Why not for life-saving treatments—and I don't mean alternative treatments (like going to Mexico). I mean drugs developed by US pharmaceutical companies that are not covered by US health insurance companies, but are covered elsewhere.

Access is one issue, but there are also different attitudes to care and even slightly different protocols with the same medications in different countries. For example, in the US, I planned to stay on Doxil until I reached the total safe cumulative dose. In the end, I did thirteen rounds of it. Had I stayed in the US, it would've gone for several more rounds, had I not recurred again during the spread-out intervals between infusions as we tried to make Doxil last for as long as possible.

When we moved to the Netherlands, doctors here said, "We'd never treat you with chemo for a year and a half straight. There's no survival advantage. The longest we'd give is six months. Then we'd repeat imaging to ensure it's working, and if you're in remission, we'd go into a watch and wait mode." You can hear from this the different attitudes, different values, different expenses that are covered (imaging, as opposed to prolonged use of chemotherapy without confirmation via imaging that it was still needed or effective).

Consider the Cost of Care

In the US in 2015, I spent $21,000 on medical expenses. The prior three years of cancer treatment, expenses were roughly equivalent. My monthly premium as a self-employed person was $802; my in-network deductible was $5,000 annually, and the out-of-network deductible was $7,500 per year.

Much to our surprise, in the Netherlands in 2016, my monthly premium for the robust plan I chose was 132 Euros per month, about five to six times lower than in the US (the conversion rate fluctuates). The annual deductible, consistent for everyone in the Netherlands, was 385 Euros in 2016. It's a system where everyone in the country, assuming they see any doctor that year, must contribute that amount to medical expenses every year beyond the affordable monthly premium. After that, everything is covered at one-hundred percent. There is no in-network or out-of-network deductible beyond that 385 Euros. And that co-insurance amount that is the same for everyone, has nothing to do with which level of insurance plan I had picked. Different plans exist, but the different levels of coverage are only reflected in different monthly premiums. For example, you can choose add-ons—supplemental coverage to fit your needs better. These include services like dental coverage, eye exams, homeopathy, physical therapy, and obstetric care. Healthcare in the Netherlands is not privatized; it is not run by the government. Instead, more than thirty companies compete to offer the best plans at the lowest prices. The care is superior to the US and the cost is much lower. Everyone is required to have insurance, and no one can be denied coverage for health insurance.

When I recurred with cancer, I didn't want to lose my hair again. I hated being bald, and it took so long to grow back. So in the US in 2014 and 2015, I paid $325 every month to rent Penguin Cold Caps, to try and keep my hair during chemo. Cumbersome, expensive, and heavy, these required a lot of work (After each use, I had to clean each of the sixteen caps and then store them in our freezer at home. A few days before each infusion, I would pack the sixteen caps in two suitcases, and then drive them to the doctor's office. They have a biomedical freezer there, which would make the caps cold enough to chill my scalp such that the chemo drugs would not stay in my hair follicles on my scalp. On chemo day, before the appointment, I'd go to the supermarket and buy fifteen pounds of dry ice. During infusion, James would don the suede work gloves, and use a laser thermometer to test each cap as he took it out of the freezer. He would need to swap the cap on my head for a new, frozen one before and every half-hour during infusion, and back at home, for a few hours after. I looked funny racing home in the car with this huge cap-thing wrapped around my head.) The caps worked; I'm very grateful for them. While I lost big tufts of hair that would come out in handfuls every time I took a shower, I had thick hair, so I still looked "normal"—you couldn't tell I was going through chemo. But what a lot of work! And that's another monthly expense.

In the Netherlands, the hospital has Paxman cap machines. One cap is fitted to your head, which has a hose that runs out the back of it. That hose gets snapped into a small knee-high height machine, which is plugged into an electrical outlet and through which very cold water circulates. When I did chemo, the nurse would wheel the machine next to the bed where I was hooked up. She'd fit the cap to my head, and plug it in. She'd turn it on, and that was all. The cap prevented hair loss and was covered by health insurance at one hundred percent.

That drug that isn't covered by my health insurance in California, olaparib, is what Dr. Barstis was trying to keep me alive to be able to use in the future. It has the potential to transform ovarian and fallopian tube cancer into a manageable disease. Yet it's not covered in the US. There is no way I could have afforded the $13,500 price tag month after month.

So while we didn't plan to immigrate to the Netherlands for financial reasons at all—it wasn't part of our equation—it has seemed like an excellent decision after the fact.

So in summary, if you're facing a major illness that is bankrupting you in the US, you might consider moving elsewhere: many countries allow you, if you're self-employed, to come as a business owner and become residents in that country. And many countries have excellent care, far better than in the US. The doctors and nurses here are as excellent as in the US, but they're not as overworked. Not nearly. I feel for doctors in the US in this age of HIPAA and electronic communications. Not only must they work all day, with only eight to sixteen or so minutes per patient to meet their quota for the insurance companies, but then they must respond to emails from patients after the workday.

Here's another example of the need for systems for border-free international healthcare in our increasingly international world: In the summer of 2014 when I was doing chemo in Los Angeles, James and I thought we'd do what we had been doing in the years before I was diagnosed, and go to Europe for three months in the summer. Dr. Barstis was in favor of our plan; he always supported me in living life as fully as possible. UCLA is part of a consortium for research with a hospital in Belgium, so he made introductions and we both went about seeing if I could do chemo there over the summer. The Belgians were helpful; the connection between doctors in LA and there was easy. But my insurance company would not cover chemotherapy there. The liaison I spoke with at my insurance company was as shocked as I was when it was denied. "Even people who are on dialysis are allowed to go on vacation!" she said. "And we cover that." She was sorry, but there was nothing she could do. I ended up flying all the way back to Los Angeles purely for a two-hour infusion. This was expensive and hard on my body. Already working hard to pay for the trip, that was an added expense, and during treatment.

In contrast to this, with any of the more than thirty Dutch insurance companies, if you request it, they mail you a card that guarantees coverage throughout the EU. In the US, I couldn't even do chemo in another state, and I had a robust, top-tier plan. (For example, I could've flown to New York or Boston from Amsterdam, rather than all the way back to Los Angeles. That would've been easier on my body, less time-consuming, and less expensive.) But the insurance company said no. So, part of being proactive and being willing to travel, means learning that there are different attitudes, different protocols, and different levels of care in different countries. You get to choose what you want. In my case, I was willing to work a little harder over the summer so that I could afford to fly back for chemo. This was the choice I preferred rather than just skipping that memorable trip.

We'll close this chapter now by sliding into the next chapter—Discernment is such an important practice, we could say it's an essential, foundational skill. Yet it's a practice that emerges from what you learn physically, emotionally, mentally and spiritually by doing your Assessment.

Another way of saying this is it is the one skill that provides the key to every area of your life. It's also the one tool that is so often lacking when we make decisions based only on our beliefs.

Discernment doesn't come naturally. Most people would rather make difficult decisions based on our values, what we long for, and hope will work, rather than evidence. In the next chapter, we'll examine why that is, and talk about how important it is (possibly a matter of life and death), to learn to discern. Then we'll learn how to practice discernment.

Thus far, we've covered the following Mental Practices in the context of the larger environmental and societal issues. We've examined how to:

Put Together Your Team;
Make a Medical Binder and Index;
Research;
Be Proactive;
Travel for Better Care;
Consider the Cost of Care.

If any of these tools draw you, write down which ones on your Menu of Practices worksheet. Or if these give you other ideas, feel free to generate your own.

Now let's consider Discernment, and discuss how you can apply this fundamental tool to every decision you face.

CHAPTER SEVENTEEN
DISCERNMENT

No problem can be solved from the same level of consciousness that created it.

\- Albert Einstein

It was long before I could believe that human learning had no clear answer to this question. For a long time it seemed to me, as I listened to the gravity and seriousness wherewith Science affirmed its positions on matters unconnected with the problem of life, that I must have misunderstood something. For a long time I was timid in the presence in learning, and I fancied that the insufficiency of the answers which I received was not its fault, but was owing to my own gross ignorance, but this thing was not a joke or a pastime with me, but the business of my life, and I was at last forced, willy-nilly, to the conclusion that these questions of mine were the only legitimate questions underlying all knowledge, and that it was not I that was in fault in putting them, but science in pretending to have an answer for them.

\- Leo Tolstoy, A Confession

Discernment

If you read only one chapter in this book, my hope for you is that you'll choose this one. Discernment has come to feel the necessary skill in navigating through nearly every challenge. And yet, we humans being the

217

creatures we are, discernment is often precisely the tool we forget to use. Or worse, it's the one in our blind spot: We think we're making sound decisions; we don't recognize our choices are based purely on our beliefs, wishes, values, or past experiences—everything but evidence. By ignoring evidence, we also dismiss our abilities to perceive accurately, to compare and judge, to assess the legitimacy of information and whether it applies to us in our unique situations. We weaken ourselves when we make decisions based solely on the beliefs or values we cling to because we believe them to be true, rather than looking at evidence; we disempower ourselves.

We all do this. Not just patients when we're anxious, who notoriously leap to conclusions, but also doctors with a conventional approach who have biases, as well as holistic practitioners with different biases than conventional doctors usually, but biases nonetheless. In all modalities, in every situation in life—it seems profoundly human to draw conclusions based on believing that what we want to believe is true. It is hard to be in the unknown; in fact, we can hardly stand it.

This is part of why there is a schism between conventional and "alternative" medicine. There's a lack of scientific literacy in laypeople, and there's a denial that science, too, can have its unspoken narrowmindedness or refusal to acknowledge other competing needs, other ways of ascertaining what is true. I'll share some examples of that below.

The moment you learn that everything you thought was true, is not true, and won't help you, inspires disappointment and rage in many. It is challenging to navigate past this threshold. Many of us simply refuse or cannot.

When we dig our heels in stubbornly this way, we are lost; we become victims of our own closed-mindedness, and we suffer as a result. To be blunt: some of us die because we cannot get beyond our beliefs.

Discernment is a skill we practice with our minds. Yet it is integrative; it calls on every aspect of us—we need insight from our physical, sensing bodies; we need to let our emotions inform our decisions, but not dictate them dogmatically; we need our intelligence to even frame the right questions, and we need a sense of purpose, meaning, or spiritual connection to make the practice of discernment worth all the trouble, at least initially.

Since being diagnosed in 2012, I've had to wake up to the fact that I was making decisions that seemed sensible and based in logic, but were not relevant ("If I just boost my immune system, it'll take care of the cancer," when in fact, the protocol to boost my immune system had no effect on the tumor marker number, so likely had no effect on the cancer.)

I needed to become aware I wasn't practicing discernment, learn how to, and remember to use it as a skill. I have found the following explanation and strategy to be the most brilliant and useful shortcut through this whole prickly mess of issues:

Ken Wilber has written a beautiful book on his wife's experiences with cancer. *In Grace and Grit: Spirituality and Healing in the Life and Death of Treya Killam Wilber*,[45] he has a chapter called, "The New Age." As Einstein suggests in the epigraph above, by observing that we need to get out of our tunnel vision and focus on the real problem at hand, Wilber describes how important it is to work with disease from the "same-level" at which disease originates, because if you do not, you create guilt or despair.

In his words:

> 1. "The standard argument from the perennial philosophy is that men and women are grounded in the Great Chain of Being. That is, we have within us matter, body, mind, soul, and spirit.
> 2. In any disease, it is extremely important to try to determine on which level or levels the disease primarily originates—physical, emotional, mental, or spiritual.
> 3. It is most important to use a 'same-level' procedure for the primary (but not necessarily sole) course of treatment. Use physical intervention for physical diseases, use emotional therapy for emotional disturbances, use spiritual methods for spiritual crises, and so on. If a mixture of causes, then use a mixture of appropriate-level treatments.
> 4. This is especially important because if you misdiagnose the disease by thinking it originates on a level higher than it in fact does, then you will generate guilt; if on a level lower, you will generate despair. Either way, the treatment will be less than effective, and will have the added disadvantage of burdening the patient with guilt or despair caused solely by the misdiagnosis."

This is so important, as so many of us cling to decisions about treatment that do not match the level at which the problem originates, and we are not even aware that's the flaw in our choice.

He continues:

> "For example, if you get hit by a bus and break a leg, that's a physical illness with physical remedies: you set the leg and plaster it. That's a 'same-level' intervention. You don't sit in the street and visualize your leg mending. That's a mental-level technique that isn't effective in this physical-level problem. Moreover, if you are told by those around you that your thoughts alone caused this accident, and that you should be able to mend the leg yourself with your thoughts, then all that is going to happen is that you will feel guilt, self-blame, and low self-esteem. It's a complete mismatch of levels and treatments.
>
> "On the other hand," he says, "if you do happen to suffer from, say, low self-esteem, because of certain scripts that you have internalized about how rotten or incompetent you are, that is a mental-level problem that responds well to a mental-level intervention such as visualization or affirmations (script rewriting, which is exactly what cognitive therapy does). Using physical-level interventions —taking megavitamins, say, or changing your diet—is not going to have much effect (unless you actually have a vitamin imbalance contributing to the problem). And if you only try to use physical-level treatments, you are going to end up in some form of despair, because the treatments are from the wrong level and they just don't work very well."[46]

These are exactly the sorts of confusions so many of us fall into. Remember my stories of the friend who was convinced if I just believed the right "things" (and ignored any "conditioned" beliefs from medicine that told me otherwise), I could cure myself of cancer, that somehow like the Lizard Boy (whose case was vague), I'd heal? Or the fellow student from healing school who, all these years later, insisted I ought to know I could simply turn off my genetic predisposition that was now being expressed in cancer? Why?

Because I taught at the healing school and "if anyone ought to know how to do that," it was [me].

These are benign, somewhat funny examples, though I allowed them to hurt my feelings at the time.

Wilber now tells the antidote:

> "So the general approach to any disease, in my opinion is to start at the bottom and work up. First, look for physical causes. Exhaust those to the best of your ability. Then move up to any possible emotional causes, and exhaust those. Then mental, then spiritual."[47]

Cancer is so widespread that you likely know, as I do, people who have adamantly refused to consider anything other than what they wanted to believe would cure them, and so died, because they made choices that do not match the level of the problem. When they didn't see improvement, they still refused to change course. The problem with cancer is that it grows; it takes over. One cannot wait forever in the hope a different-level intervention will work, even if we wish it would. Even if it makes sense to our value system that it should be efficacious.

Wilber clarifies when it's useful to choose treatments from other levels:

> "Now this is not to say that treatments from other levels can't be very important in a supporting or adjuvant fashion. They most definitely can. In the simple example of the broken leg, relaxation techniques, visualization, affirmations, meditation, psychotherapy if you need it—all of those can contribute to a more balanced atmosphere in which physical healing can more easily and perhaps readily occur.

> "What is not helpful is taking the fact that these psychological and spiritual aspects can be very useful, and then saying that the reason you broke your leg is that you lacked these psychological and spiritual facets in the first place. A person suffering any major illness may make significant and profound changes in the face of that illness; it does not follow that they got the illness because they lacked the changes. That would be like saying, if you have a fever

and you take aspirin the fever goes down; therefore having a fever is due to an aspirin deficiency."

So we can utilize all the other helpful tools that we believe are useful (think of the friend with breast cancer, sad and disappointed about her divorce, who began to do emotional work around her relationships). The challenge lies in realizing that while that work is beneficial emotionally, it is not from the right level to affect the physical issue of cancer. To believe otherwise is dangerous, to be convinced otherwise, for example by people around you, is misleading.

And yet: Wilber's final point speaks to the premises of energy healing and the synergistic possibilities touched on with this TTC Method (that we need research to confirm). He puts it this way:

> "Now most diseases, of course, don't originate from a single and isolated level. Whatever happens on one level or dimension of being affects all the other levels to a greater or lesser degree. One's emotional, mental, and spiritual makeup can most definitely influence physical illness and physical healing, just as a physical illness can have strong repercussions on the higher levels. Break your leg, and it will probably have emotional and psychological effects. In systems theory this is called 'upward causation'—a lower level is causing certain events in a higher level. And the reverse, 'downward causation,' is when a higher level has a causal effect or influence on the lower.
>
> "The question, then, is just how much 'downward causation' does the mind—do our thoughts and emotions—have on physical illness? And the answer seems to be: much more than was once thought, not nearly as much as new agers believe."[46]

Wilber then goes on to discuss psychoneuroimmunology. While this book of his was published in 2001, we've learned a great deal more in the intervening years about the effects our beliefs and emotions have on the physical body—remember the woman going through ovarian cancer who feels lonely despite her friends and family wanting to be there for her? We know that her perceived loneliness affects gene expression, which modulates the flow of the hormone cascade and the release of particular neuropeptides; these cause her cancer to recur earlier and metastasize more widely, as we discussed. We also know that feelings of loneliness affect the blood chemistry for eighty days. So we can do the emotional work—we can prescribe, "Get some new friends! It'll aid your survival." But we must not fall asleep and believe that doing so, or working with our emotions, is sufficient to cure cancer once it has started; it's contrary to evidence to insist it can. And such insistence leads to guilt and despair. Maintained as a final position for too long, it can be life-threatening.

At the same time, it is useful to enlist our beliefs, feelings, and emotions to check in with ourselves and make choices that affect the quality of our lives. Quality of life is an important distinction from cure, and one which will likely grow in importance as survival rates improve and cancer becomes a manageable disease. Use of our mind-body connection to improve quality of life is not dangerous, but rather useful.

So what does discernment look like and how do we practice it?

Discernment Means Distinguish and Choose

At core, you want to be aware of all your options, and distinguish between what is helpful and what harmful. You do not want to close your eyes and make decisions based only on hope or what seems sensible (but has no supporting evidence). Rather, you want to make smart choices in ways that make sense to you and call on all your ways of knowing what is right for you—physically, emotionally, mentally, and spiritually. You want to practice discernment pragmatically for diagnosis, assessment, care and the quality of your life, meaning, how it feels to be alive. Discernment is another stage of development after the "rose-colored glasses" phase of just deciding from a naive, suggestible point of view. Here are some potential questions to ask, possible areas to distinguish:

• Does it work? The most important question, and the one we usually don't ask. Variations include: Is it efficacious? Is it working for me? Sometimes a regimen works, and then stops working; other times it works for others, but not you. Occasionally, it may work for you even though it doesn't work for others. We don't know enough about this yet—why what works for some doesn't work for others. But by asking this question and staying awake to the shifting landscape of whether something is working, you can craft the best life possible.

• How can you assess if your choices are working? There are diagnostic tools (imaging, blood work, biopsies, genomic assessment of tissue samples, etcetera), and there are treatment tools. If you choose an "alternative" treatment, you can still use conventional medical tools to diagnose and assess if your treatment of choice is working.

• What's helpful and what's harmful? Know that these are often conditioned by our beliefs. One person may have had negative experiences with conventional medicine in the past, and so now is unwilling or unable to consider using it. Another person may have religious beliefs that affect how one answers this question. Deciding what's helpful and what's harmful is a personal decision, but sometimes, if you're awake about it, you can catch yourself in the act of drawing conclusions based on past experiences. Then you can choose if that decision fits you now or is merely a red flag, a marker alerting you to a need—then you can get what you need to make the new possible choice work for you. For example, I have a friend who has a treatable thyroid cancer now. She's had so many negative experiences with allopathic doctors in her past serious medical issues, that she is not willing right now to consider conventional medical treatment. I could say, "Just treat it conventionally. Conventional treatment works for this kind of cancer. It's an easy cancer; you can be all done and well in just a few weeks," but that's not helpful to her. It disempowers her and discounts her feelings. A more useful set of questions might be, "If you know this is treatable, what would you need to make treating it conventionally feel good for you? Do you need a doctor you can really talk to and trust, with whom you can share your past experiences? Do you need to know others' experiences on Synthroid or natural hormones? Or are you set—have you made up your mind and now just want my support for the choice you've already made?" Often people cannot get to the underlying need, because they don't know how. So they get stuck at an absolute position because they don't have a way to ask themselves if they're making decisions based on defense or past experiences, as my friend has sometimes been able to articulate in this example. This TTC Method aims to help get to the underlying need and then get that need met. By getting the need met, the upward and downward causation that Wilber describes also gets addressed: the person can make a choice for a physical treatment, and by communicating what's needed to make that a choice one is willing to make, one also addresses the emotional issue ("I've had bad experiences with conventional medicine," or "I don't like doctors,") and the mental beliefs, ("I'll have the same negative experience again.") By challenging one's beliefs, one gets to heal those as well, and have a new, more positive experience.

• What's unique about your case/biology/histology? Based on knowing your unique situation or cell type, for example, what's called for in your situation? For example, I know someone who tried a raw food diet and it worked for her—she's still alive years later. For me, my tumor marker kept increasing while on the same diet. Was that because the tumor in my body was caused by gene expression that does not respond to a raw food diet? Was it because the tumor was estrogen receptor positive? We don't know. But each person/cell type/histology is unique. Honor that and you'll have more success. Dig your heels in and insist what works for others must work similarly for you, and you're setting yourself up at the very least for disappointment; at worst, it could be life-threatening.

• How much time can you take before you must decide? That, too, varies, but is worth learning so you have clarity and peace of mind.

• Who is a worthy member of your team—in other words, who is a "quack" and who can help? Ask to see results, not just beliefs. Most practitioners keep track of what results they're getting. At my request, the doctor I ended up switching away from put me in touch with a few "long-term" survivors. There were only three of them; they've all since died. My discomfort with her was for other reasons, but the doctors I switched to have better outcomes.

• Do the qualities of your practitioner feel good to you or not? What qualities do you want in each doctor/therapist/healer?

• Are you choosing what you want or what others want you to do?

- These are just jumping off places. Feel free to add your own. The main trick is to try and observe yourself using your beliefs to make decisions, and then ask these questions to get to the core issues. Then use all your skills—physical, emotional, mental, and spiritual—to discern.

How Do We Practice Discernment?

We practice discernment by using the tools of our Assessment. That is, we scan our bodies and notice, what's happening physically, emotionally, mentally and spiritually. What do we need? If you work the Self-Tracking and Tracking Other with a partner, what gets uncovered there—can your partner/therapist/healer/nurse notice where you fall into blind spots? Can this person gently, with respect, ask you questions so you can clarify your views and decide if you want to stay in your current position? Can your practitioner resonate with you so you can drop into your true feelings and so get to your need underlying a (perhaps defensive) initial choice?

Once your Assessment reveals your true needs, how can you meet those needs? Discernment can help you choose among competing potential choices.

Let's look at how this plays out. We'll consider some of the common issues that come up around questions of discernment.

Lack of Dialogue Between Specialties

In 2012, when I was initially diagnosed with cancer, my primary care physician was a functional medicine doctor. I liked her a lot. She is smart, funny, caring, and good at "connecting the dots" in patients' health histories: She'd take a detailed history, order blood and urine tests, and based on the results, that would reveal what needed to be treated. The treatment consisted of prescription-strength supplements which I could buy in her office. These seemed helpful for a range of issues, and I liked the idea of supplements—it felt like they were less likely than pharmaceutical medicines to cause side effects or harm me, because they are "natural." (You can hear my bias there. I'm a healer. Supplements went along with my value system.) This doctor also monitored me for cancer, so it was she who called that day to tell me my CA-125 tumor marker was elevated. She also referred me to my first surgeon.

She is an MD, and a fine practitioner. The problem arose in the schism between the functional medicine she practiced and the conventional hematology-oncology practiced by my then new chemo doctor.

To make a very long story short, as I began treatment, I also began supplements that my trusted functional MD prescribed. Within one round of chemo, I was anemic. We had to postpone the second round. The hematologist-oncologist said, "You're healthy overall. Something's wrong. You shouldn't be anemic yet. What are you taking?"

James and I literally drove from that appointment to my functional medicine doctor's office, and we waited for her to squeeze me in between appointments. "It's not the supplements that are 'bad,' and making you anemic," she said. "It's the chemo." We went back to the chemo doc.: "It's the supplements." No one could tell me what was going on or what to do about it. We couldn't safely keep postponing chemo or the cancer would almost certainly grow back after surgery; the tumor marker was already creeping back up. I had already delayed chemo for a few weeks anyway when I went to MD Anderson to get that second opinion. In the midst of all this back and forth, I called the pharmacist at MD Anderson, then a man named Jack Watkins. He was the first and only person in the country it seemed who could explain to me what was happening. The supplements contained ingredients that were metabolized by a certain enzyme, called cytochrome P450, and this was the same pathway that cleared the chemo from my liver.[49] Because the chemo couldn't be cleared, it was staying in my body longer than normal and killing more healthy cells than normal. Hence I was anemic.

This was my first exposure of many to the lack of dialogue between different approaches to the practice of medicine.

I had to surrender my belief that the supplements were helpful in that situation. I had to accept the fact that these two styles of practitioners, while both MDs, had their own biases, and neither could explain definitively how and why these medications interacted. I was shocked it was so hard to find anyone who knew what was going on.

Something Seems Logical or Sensible, But Is Not Efficacious, or Not Efficacious for You

In the section on the Assessment to Foster Discernment, I shared about my attempts to try a raw food diet and wheatgrass juicing. As I mentioned just above, it agreed with my value system to think, "I'll just boost my immune system, and that'll take care of the cancer." (You can hear how I mixed levels there, not so much in terms of the actual regimen, but in terms of my mental belief that it would affect the physical.) That logic for the protocol to work seems sensible, and I felt and looked great while juicing that much—as I said, my skin was radiant, my hair was shiny. But it had no effect. When the president of that organization insisted, "You don't really have cancer," as I mentioned, it was so tempting to be seduced, to "fall asleep" and believe him. My friend did. But the diagnostic assessment in the form of the rising marker made the need for discernment obvious: this regimen did not work for me. Even though it would have been tempting to say "just give it more time." Even though it seemed like it should, and even though the claim seemed sensible (our immune systems fight disease all the time—why not bolster it)?, the reality was it had no effect for me. And most important: I didn't have the luxury of time to keep trying it.

I asked Dr. Friedman about discernment, and he said: "Patients are being offered what they want—a treatment that doesn't make them feel sick and doesn't feel like medication or part of industrial health. People tend not to question things they find appealing and want to do."

He's a surgeon, so I asked him how he copes with this, or if it feels like he's fighting an uphill battle. "If I do the best job I can do," he said, "I feel good about it. Plenty of patients I've had over the years do things I think are crazy. I'll keep treating them if they'll let us. I respect people's right of self-determination. I know some battles we'll win and some we'll never win. What we do is inform people what the consequences of their decisions will be. People need to have the right to do that."

I asked him how that plays out in his practice, and he gave this example: "A woman in her mid-thirties declined chemo for her ovarian cancer. She believed if God wanted her, God could take her. How do you answer that? I offered her chemo. But at the time she was diagnosed, she probably had stage one disease. Three months later, it had grown back all over her abdomen. You have to let people make their own decision. Our healthcare system is based on consent. I can't force anybody to do what they don't want to do."

How Much Time Do You Have to Make Up Your Mind?

When I asked Dr. Chrysopoulo, my breast surgeon, about these questions of discernment, he had this to say about choosing your team. I asked him if there were qualities in doctors that he thinks patients could learn to look for. He said:

"Not holding back. Not just going with the first thing they hear. You want patients to get their questions answered and feel as comfortable as possible. Doctors are human. Human nature dictates that we push things we're most comfortable with. Physicians are also in potentially abusive dynamics." I asked what he meant, and he said, "You can sway opinions. You can give two patients exactly the same information, with the same diagnosis. And just by way you deliver it, you can get two patients to do two different things. I'm not saying doctors do so on purpose. But we have the power to do that. We need to recognize that, and use it in the right way, and not abuse it. Be cognizant of the fact that doctors are human. I don't mean by going on message boards. You need to weed out the quackery and the good info. Unfortunately, when you have a cancer diagnosis, everything is an emergency. You did it—right? Cancer patients do have a little bit of time. Do you have six months to do your research? Probably not. Tomorrow or a month isn't going to make or break you in most cases."

I asked him to clarify, as this was the most concrete I had ever heard for how much time a patient can take to make up her mind about what she wants. He was discussing breast cancer, because he does mastectomies and reconstructions, and he said,

"You want it taken care of within six weeks from diagnosis. We know that. If you're not getting a response to your questions, find answers to them elsewhere. Only doctors uncomfortable with their opinion frown on second opinions. Because if that patient chooses to go with the second opinion, that patient probably wouldn't have been happy with your care—it's not a fit for some reason."

He reiterated that he likes to work where there's a feeling of shared decision making with the patient.

I asked him specifically which discerning questions he would recommend patients ask. He answered,

"We feel pressured every day. Many other specialties feel pressured every day especially when it comes to cancer care, prolonging life. I find it interesting that not many patients ask the physician if they would sign up for that same treatment. That's a different question than 'What would you do if I was your wife?' It's a different answer than 'What would you do if you were me?'" "Quite frankly," he continued, "if my wife had pancreatic cancer, and it wasn't caught very early, I probably would want to do everything. It's my wife, I'd want to do everything. I'm a physician. I know survival is diabolical. She'd want to do everything because of our daughters, and I'd support that. But if it were me, I don't want to do everything. No chemo. Just make sure I don't have pain. I'd want to go where we went on our honeymoon. Get one last trip in. It's hard to be a doctor because of what we know—we know the failings of medicine, where things fall short, the futility of some of them. We succumb to family pressures though we know what the likelihood is, but deep down you know it's not going to be good. Would you sign up for that if it was you? That's what I struggle with—the breast cancer patient we could be getting has a chance with conventional treatment, but chooses to go with a completely raw diet. All you can do is tell them, explain to them, and respect their choice."

I agree with this, and I'm interested in the fact that both Dr. Friedman and Dr. Chrysopoulo articulated the same ethos. And I believe it's acceptable to offer the possibility, through these questions, to consider the choice. If the client/patient has decided, then it's obviously only appropriate at that point to support her or him in that decision. If she or he is struggling to decide, you can share information, yes, and you can share this "meta" perspective through the Assessment tool and the practice of Discernment. Both tools open a doorway into the patient really knowing her or himself—not just in a state of panic, but slowly, gently, patiently. Then if she or he makes the same choice, it will have a peaceful quality to it, like she or he is aware of the risks and knows inside this is the right decision. If she or he ends up changing and making a new choice, that, too, will be the result of this process of coming to know one's deep, true needs.

CHAPTER EIGHTEEN
SPIRITUAL PRACTICES

Can I get used to it day after day
a little at a time while the tide keeps
coming in faster the waves get bigger
building on each other breaking records
this is not the world that I remember
then comes the day when I open the box
that I remember packing with such care
and there is the face that I had known well
in little pieces staring up at me
it is not mentioned on the front pages
but somewhere far back near the real estate
among the things that happen every day
to someone who now happens to be me
and what can I do and who can tell me
then there is what the doctor comes to say
endless patience will never be enough
the only hope is to be the daylight

- W.S. Merwin, "Living with the News"

Spiritual Practices

Have you ever been to a play, or read a book, and you find that it speaks to the state you're in? When I was in college, I would notice that my response to anything I read had a lot to do with what mood I was in when I read it. That seemed curious as this was right at the advent of postmodernism and the transition from believing in collective "Truth" with a capital "T" to a subsequent belief that truth is relative. When I started college we were taught to write as objectively as possible and keep our own responses out of our theses. Four years later, the belief in the objectivity of the narrator was over—now we were instructed to include ourselves in the writing. I found this challenging, as there was no single "self" I could describe—my feelings vacillated all the time.

This sense of being outside myself observing has stayed with me. If I get immersed in a really good book, I enter the world of the characters and relax into the feeling of being in that world, rather than the one I'm actually in. That's one of the great joys of reading, and I'm not the only one who describes it this way: I lose track of time and don't think of anything else. Another way of saying this is, reading changes my state. This changing of our individual inner states interests me.

Something similar happens often when I go to concerts. James loves classical music, especially piano pieces. We've heard many of the great pianists performing today. Unlike James, I don't learn as well aurally. As a result, often I find, on any given night when we're planning to go to a concert, that I get engrossed in my work and beforehand get cranky. It's hard to stop what I'm doing, and I inevitably feel, "I'm too busy and don't have time to go." Then I get dressed up, and in Amsterdam we travel everywhere by bicycle. It's often cold out, and as we ride to the Concertgebouw hall, I start to relax. The more wound up I am before the concert, the more the transition changes my state. By the time we're seated and the musician makes his entrance, I'm happy, in the flow, glad to be with James and any friends we've arranged to meet there, content that I stepped away from my work.

But then the magic happens. Sometimes if the pianist is exceptional, from the first note, something shifts inside me. It sends a little shiver of recognition through me. James and I look at each other, because we've each felt it; we've both recognized it. This is what we've come for: transcendence. And as the music swells, the whole audience is enwrapped together. Without consciously noticing, we synchronize our breathing. We become a coherent body. We are no longer hundreds of separate people, mired in the mundane concerns of ordinary life, but lifted, together, to some exalted place. By the encore, we are washed up on some other shore, refreshed, transformed, returned to our individuality, but still full of the good feeling of being a human being among other human beings, in a building that resonates and has been holding and conducting sound for centuries.

It's the same with emails, believe it or not. I am always curious about the fact that the state I'm in when I draft an email seems to affect the response I get. It's mysterious to me, as if some energetic transmission happens through the ether, and the personality concerns of the humans communicating comes through, too. Maybe someday we'll understand.

And maybe that understanding will have something to do with knowing how energy healing works, too.

I practice healing, and I have studied, read, thought, and written about it for decades; you might say I've devoted my life to it. But I do not understand it, and I cannot explain how it works. How do my clients not in the same room with me experience and describe, with such precision, exactly what I'm doing during a healing session? If I'm in Amsterdam, say, and my client is in Melbourne, Australia, at the end of the healing session when we talk by phone again, she's likely to say something like, "I could really feel you working on those little bones at the base of my skull, the ones behind my head at the top of my neck where I was having pain. I forgot to tell you about it. But you were working there, weren't you? What were you doing?" And I marvel because I was working exactly there, on her occipital bones; I cleared old tension and fear stored there. How could I perceive, accurately apparently, that that's what is held there, and how could she feel that's what I was doing? This is not a rare experience; it happens with almost every client in every session. It happens whether or not they "believe in" energy healing.

Skype has made the exploration into this subject of what is the transmission of energy even more fascinating. Sometimes in a Skype session, the client likes to stay connected during the whole appointment. So he'll call me at the scheduled time, we'll talk for a few minutes, and then he may go lie down on his couch in his living room, for example, in Brooklyn, as one example. I can pivot my computer so the camera faces the massage table in my office. I give the healing as if he's in the room with me. I can see him on his couch in his apartment, and, if he opens his eyes, he can see me standing and "working on him" as if he's on the massage table in the same room with me in Amsterdam. Typically as the healing gets underway, we both close our eyes. He may fall asleep or just drift into a state of deep relaxation. Meanwhile, I'm sensing him—checking every level, working where my perceptions draw me. I feel energy running through my hands, and they become hot. The amount of flow seems to be something I can modulate as I sense how much the client needs and how much gets pushed back towards me like backwash. Sometimes, a jolt of energy passes through me, and in those times, what shocks me most is I'll open my eyes at the moment of the jolt, and look at the computer screen to make sure my client is all right. Typically, his body will twitch in that moment, as though the jolt of energy just went through him at what may be a split-second after I felt it. I don't know how to explain this. Maybe someday we'll understand.

For now, knowing this, I make sure I'm in the state I want to be in when I give healings, just as I do when I send that email. When I give healings, I make sure I'm in a clear, charged and balanced state, to the best of my ability. How do I do that? Through practices, including the ones we've learned here in this book.

I'm curious about the notion that if that state we're in affects our experience, it may affect gene expression, too.

For me, what I do not yet understand, but have direct experience of, begins to touch on the spiritual. Here are some spiritual practices which may have beneficial effects on health.

Meditation

There are different kinds of meditation, which, it appears, create different physiological, emotional and spiritual effects. There are many medical studies which confirm the benefits of most kinds of meditation. You can choose which style has the potential to give the benefits you want, and practice regularly. You might consider mantra meditation, in which you repeat a certain word or sound, usually considered a sacred vibration in the language (often Sanskrit) in which that style of meditation was developed and refined. You can practice mindfulness meditation, in which you bring your attention to the present moment, again and again, nonjudgmentally. You can practice vipassana meditation, and focus on the breath, or gaze at a candle flame. When your mind wanders, you bring it back to what you are focusing on. You can meditate while contemplating sacred art, like a thangka or a mandala. You might consider practicing chakra meditation, and let your voice make the different vowel sounds that correspond to the frequencies of each chakra, as described in this book, and much more extensively elsewhere. These are just a few examples.

When I asked Dr. Cole, the social genomics researcher at UCLA, about the possible effects of meditation on the genome, he had this to say:

"There's not one style of meditation; for example mindfulness is not necessarily better than mantra meditation. What's important is not the one way people get there, but the fact that they get there and do feel different.

There are likely many ways to get there. And this feeling definitely affects one's quality of life. But a eudaimonic feeling that it's not all about oneself, but rather being of service to others, does appear to be key."[50] Let's now dig in to what he means by this "eudaimonic feeling."

Meaning-Making: The Eudaimonic vs. The Hedonic

We humans have a need for meaning. Many of us may no longer feel the comfort of believing in traditional religious explanations, and as a result may no longer have answers to our spiritual questions. We may live in a time in which many of us in the West no longer practice organized religion. Yet we can, and find we do, still craft meaning, because we realize we need it. Just as we love because we need to, we make meaning because we seem to be hardwired for it. It soothes us to not feel so powerless and as though the rough, raw aspects of life are completely beyond our control.

Some of us who no longer believe in the customs and rituals of our religions as practiced by our ancestors, still long for community. So we get involved with various new groups that meet the same needs as a congregation did in the past. Others actively make new rituals and create new ceremonies. (I'm always amused by how many Dutch people attend classical music concerts on Sunday afternoons. I think I'm not the only one who gets that oceanic feeling at concerts. In this historically Calvinist country, it seems music has replaced church.)

Part of why we make meaning is what Dr. Cole described as the distinction between the eudaimonic and the hedonic. These two forms of well-being or happiness have been debated and discussed by philosophers dating back at least to Aristotle. Hedonic happiness is based on self-gratification and avoidance of pain. Eudaimonic well-being is based on a sense of meaning and self-realization. It turns out that our bodies recognize the difference: Remember the woman with ovarian cancer who feels lonely and that affects her gene expression, which in turn directly affects her cancer? Dr. Cole and Barbara Fredrickson, PhD, a psychologist at University of North Carolina at Chapel Hill, set out to see if ongoing positive experiences would have the opposite result as loneliness on the genome. We already knew from prior studies that eudaimonic and hedonic aspects of well-being had been linked to longevity, so it seemed plausible that there might be a beneficial effect. They expected that hedonic self-gratification as a form of happiness would show up on the genome more than some notion that one needs a sense of purpose and meaning in life. But much to their surprise, the opposite showed. Hedonically-happy people didn't register on the genome, but people high in eudaimonic happiness were more likely to show the opposite gene expression compared to those who were lonely: Specifically— antiviral response increased and inflammation decreased. There have been three replications of the study since 2013, and Dr. Cole says that the data suggest that lacking a sense of meaning and purpose can be as damaging as obesity or smoking.[51]

Remember when we discussed Grotowski's idea of the expressive body versus the trained body? Just like making meaning, we express (that is, we enjoy being our true selves rather than simply compliant to others' wishes of how we should be), because we like the feeling of being who we really are. We respond to that vitality in each other because we recognize that much aliveness; we like being around people who are vibrantly, unapologetically themselves. We like it because we fundamentally want access to all of ourselves. Many of us human beings lose the thread of connection with ourselves, however. Life gets busy, we fall into roles or mundane tasks of living. Illness has the potential to call us out of that slumber. It's a foundational human longing to want to keep growing, to want access to our full selves, both in how we live in relationship with ourselves as well as in relationship with each other. That gives our lives meaning. Knowing this, you can, if you want, choose to use your illness for your own development, as a way to access more and more of your true (not tamed) self. You then are using your illness for your own self-realization.

This is what Dr. Asher meant when he co-designed his GRACE program to talk about legacy creation. It's not that the program solely spotlights death, but focusing on one's legacy lets people live a fuller life. When you consider what you want to be known for, and which values are most important to you, that allows you to live that way now. The passions that you share with those around you—that's part of how we make meaning.

Compassion and Oneness

I often think of Saint Augustine. He happened to live "in interesting times," as we do today. A wild playboy in his youth, he converted to Christianity at age thirty-one, influenced Catholic theology, and wrote books we still read today. He, too, thought about the mind-body-soul connection. At the end of his life, his city, Hippo, was overrun by an invading army, the

Vandals. When I read him in college we learned that he died as a result of being trampled by an elephant as the army stormed the town. Now, I cannot find any mention of that dramatic story online. All accounts say that during the summer of the invasion, he got sick, and he died within days. Still, all of his wisdom, his spiritual growth, all his self-actualization, and then...it was over, for him personally, and the people in his city, who reverted back to a more primitive, warring way of living.

His time sounds familiar.

So, thinking back to the beginning of the book, where we explored the need for the Thriving Through Cancer Method, when we discussed how overwhelming it can sometimes seem to live in the "interesting times" of today, the question, from a spiritual perspective is: Can you be one with everything and everyone—the refugees, the suicide bombers, the leaders, the public? Think about it: How did your family get to where they live now? My family walked out of Russia to escape the pogroms. That's not so different from the refugees of today. The suicide bombers? I, too, remember being a teenager who wanted to change the world and make it what I believed was better. I, too, wanted a cause to believe in, something that promised to make my life worthwhile, larger than ordinary life. I wanted to transform adulthood away from the mundane demands of just earning a living to something that warranted all the hoopla. And I, too, wanted to achieve that grand undertaking via some community that would require me to give everything over from my individual self to the ideology for the sake of the group. The political leaders? They are not alone. I, too, think of policy and how to make life as good as possible for the greatest number of people. The public? Sometimes, I, too, am overwhelmed, and just want to be left alone or sink into angry judgment of others. Really, in all these cases, I can empathize with the people involved. More than that, I can identify with each person's point of view. See what this is like for you: the cliche of "we are each other" starts to feel literally true.

Now look again at your Menu of Practices on the worksheet in the Appendix. What are your spiritual needs, and do any of these practices feel like they serve you? We've covered:

Meditation;

Meaning-Making; and

Compassion and Oneness.

The first time I had cancer in 2012, doing chemo was challenging. As the treatment wore on, the cancer cells were being killed, yes, but I was also getting weaker and sicker. By the fifth round of six, the edge of what I think of as me was clearly dissolving: I had blood in one eye from broken blood vessels, I kept getting a bloody nose, an abscess formed on my skin, I could not breathe deeply from the anemia—it seemed like I was bleeding from every orifice. It was such a strange feeling. The Carboplatin in Carbo-Taxol is made from platinum, which came to earth from supernovas. As the drugs coursed through my veins, it started to feel like the phrase "we are star stuff" was literally true, and the old alchemical phrase "as above, so below" could be rephrased as, "as within, so without." Sometimes it seemed like there was no edge of me; like there ceased to be any distinction between the cells which composed my body and the cosmos.

And what is cancer if not unbridled, untrammeled, free, runaway growth? If we are in the habit of communicating with the consciousness of our cells, we could argue that cancer cells are "confused," but it is part of human nature to be curious, to grow, to want to know more, just like the expressive body versus the tamed body Grotowski describes. We could look at the Garden of Eden story the same way. Adam and Eve just wanted to know. So they ate from the Tree of Knowledge.

Over the years, in times when I would feel the most frightened and sad if I felt I was dying, I would talk with my therapist, Michael Mervosh. I knew him through the healing school. Initially he was one of the teachers there, then when I joined the faculty, we were colleagues. Later he became my therapist. After all these years of knowing each other in different contexts, I could really dig in and talk frankly with him about all my feelings about dying. A psychologist and energy healer by training, he is a wise man. Deeply embodied, present, able to resonate, and affecting the lives of hundreds of people in the many programs he has created in which he now teaches, Michael would say, "Each person needs to come to a place of acceptance." And, "Acceptance is not the same as resignation." When I asked him how he felt about dying, he said that at death he "wants to be one drop in the ocean of life that merges with other drops." And, "Surrender is not the same as submission."

I sense what he means. From this perspective, it doesn't matter what we accomplish, or how much we get done. It isn't even sad that we get so attached to our lives, and then we die. It just is. We live and we die.

So, now, contemplate that: From this perspective, this vantage point, it doesn't matter how long we live. It matters how we live.

Live congruently with how you want to live.

EPILOGUE

--

GENETICS AND EPIGENETICS

EPILOGUE
GENETICS AND EPIGENETICS
AND THE MEDICINE
OF THE FUTURE

5

What is it then between us?
What is the count of the scores or hundreds of years between us?

Whatever it is, it avails not—distance avails not, and place
avails not,
I too lived, Brooklyn of ample hills was mine,
I too walk'd the street of Manhattan island, and bathed in
the waters around it,
I too felt the curious abrupt questionings stir within me,
In the day among crowds of people sometimes they came upon me,
In my walks home late at night or as I lay in my bed they
came upon me,
I too had been struck from the float forever held in solution,
I too had received identity by my body,
That I was I knew was of my body, and what I should be I
knew I should be of my body.

7

Closer yet I approach you,
What thought you have of me now, I had as much of you—I
Laid my stores in advance,
I consider'd long and seriously of you before you were born.

Who was to know what should come home to me?
Who knows but I am enjoying this?
Who knows, for all the distance, but I am as good as looking
at you now, for all you cannot see me?

- Walt Whitman, "Crossing Brooklyn Ferry"

We began this book with my personal medical history—the story of my first breast biopsy in 1997, that happened to correspond to the early days of genetic testing for the BRCA mutation. In the nineteen years since, I was healthy for fifteen years, until 2012, when my gene must have "turned on"—I was diagnosed with fallopian tube cancer. I have survived longer than statistics suggest would be likely. Despite three recurrences (including five surgeries, twenty-three rounds of chemo, and eighteen radiotherapy treatments to date), I am alive, once again in remission, and I feel well. I'm living a full life.

My health history over these past nineteen years has also paralleled the story of mapping the human genome (at least the euchromatic regions—the heterochromatic regions, found in centromeres and telomeres—have not yet been sequenced; they may end up being more important than we realize).

Since crossing the key dates of the human genome project (starting with the year 2000, when the draft sequence was announced, then the completion of the sequencing in 2003, and then the sequence of the last chromosome, in 2006), we are now in a full-blown metamorphosis in medicine. Known as the genomic revolution, we now have new understandings of human evolution, how species interact with and adapt to new environments, and how cancer cells respond to drugs. We are already seeing translation of data both to conceptions of how cancer and other diseases work and new ways to treat these fatal illnesses—all based on new understandings of our genes. The model of how to conduct research is also changing, to collaborative methods and data sharing, which is also a radical phenomenon.

There is still much we do not know, and I don't know whether these advances will come soon enough to keep me alive, but they really may. Here is what we do know. We'll look at three areas: Genetics, epigenetics, and what we've been exploring throughout this book—the possibility that mind-body connection can be developed in part to influence health.

Genetics

There are five interrelated new ways to treat cancer we'll look at here that are emerging from our still developing understanding of the human genome:
- Genomic Assessment;
- Targeted Therapy;
- Immunotherapy;
- CRISPR (Clustered Regularly Interspersed Short Palindromic Repeats)-Cas9
- Mind-Body Attempts to Influence Gene Expression

Genomic assessment is a test to see which genetic mutations are present in a tumor. Based on this information, it is easier to know which drugs are likely to be efficacious. Further, by knowing and indexing which genetic mutations show up in a particular tissue sample, drugs developed in the future can be matched with patients most likely to benefit. (And somewhat cynically, I wonder if pharmaceutical companies will have access to the database, too, and so know which genes are being expressed in large numbers of tumors, and therefore know what the "market," in this case patients, needs, therefore which research should be prioritized in order to maximize profits.) Still, cynicism aside, it's amazing that a sample just a few millimeters thick can be examined and matched to the most efficacious drugs.

Targeted Therapy

Essentially, whether or not someone has a genetic predisposition, all cancer begins when specific genes in healthy cells mutate. Targeted therapy drugs do not kill cancer cells like traditional chemo medications. Instead, they target specific proteins or genes in or on the surface of cancer cells. These proteins send signals that tell the cancer cells to either grow and divide, make new blood vessels, prevent cell death, or keep cells living longer than normal. By targeting these proteins, the cancer cells cannot carry out their tasks that would result in their growth and spread. Targeted therapy is the foundation of precision medicine, the new concept of tailoring treatment to each patient based on which genes or proteins are present in the cancer.

Immunotherapy

Bolstering the immune system so it can do the job of fighting cancer has historically seemed like a strategy that ought to work, and over the decades, many attempts have been made in this direction.[52] The alternative protocol I tried that had no effect for me, was an attempt to bolster my immune system through raw food and wheatgrass juicing. My disappointing experience was hardly unique—historically, immunotherapy has only worked for a minority of patients in only a limited range cancer types.

Yet the field of immunotherapy is evolving rapidly: Researchers investigating how the immune system recognizes tumors, have started to understand what, exactly, is being recognized. Just since March 2016, researchers have published evidence that as a tumor develops, its genetic faults, known as antigens, can be flagged on the surface of a cancer cell. The tumor knows how to switch off the immune system so it doesn't recognize the cancerous cells. But by knowing the tumor cells' genetic signature, like a red flag, the T-cells of the immune system can be activated to recognize that flag, and target all the tumor cells at once. In the future, drugs or a therapeutic vaccine could be developed to activate T-cells or harvest, grow, and administer T-cells that recognize the antigens back into the patient. This takes the new notion of precision medicine to an even more personalized level—treatments would be "bespoke," made for each patient based on the antigens expressed by that patient's unique cancer cells.[53]

CRISPR-Cas9

Clustered Regularly Interspersed Short Palindromic Repeats or more commonly known by its acronym, CRISPR, is shorthand for a way to "cut and paste" genes. It naturally occurs in bacteria as a way that they defend against viruses. Since the discovery of CRISPR at three different institutions between 1987 and 1997, and since its presentation at conferences starting in 2000, it is gaining widespread application in research. Since it has been discovered as naturally occurring, researchers are quickly beginning to use it: Between 2012 and the present, it has been recognized that the combination of CRISPR system with Cas9 protein can be deliberately "told" where to "cut" via guide RNA. In 2013, researchers fused two RNA molecules into a "single-guide RNA" that, when mixed with Cas9, could find and cut the DNA target specified by the guide RNA. The Cas9 system could be "told" to target any sequence in DNA and "cut" it—this is accomplished by manipulating the nucleotide sequence of the guide RNA. As a result, research is rapidly progressing in editing genomes with the reengineered CRISPR-Cas9 system. It has been used in a wide range of organisms, including baker's yeast, zebrafish, fruit flies, axolotls (Mexican salamanders), nematodes (roundworms), plants, mice, monkeys, and human embryos. The potential is that one day we will be able to "cut" out a tumor suppressor gene like the BRCA1 gene, and "paste" in a healthy gene. Already, the making of mice genetically-engineered to have or lack particular genes is gaining popularity as a result of CRISPR-Cas9.[54] And in June 2016, a ten-year extension of the human genome project was announced in the form of a new project—HGP-Write—that is, the human genome project to *synthesize* the human genome.[55] Not yet sponsored by any government, it is still beginning, despite ethical debates.

What do these new approaches look like clinically? Soon it may no longer be relevant to follow treatment protocols originally developed according to which primary cancer one has—in other words, where the cancer originated in the body (i.e, breast cancer, ovarian cancer, renal cancer, etcetera. When cancer recurs or metastasizes, we still consider it the original type of cancer it was the first time, even though that body part may have been removed surgically.) But as we develop these new, targeted therapies, the key information is which protein is the "lock" that fits the "key" of the drug. Dr. Barstis spoke about what that looks like with a patient, this way:

> "Now in genomic assessment, every cancer is an individual cancer. We're beginning to understand why and we can use precision medicine."
>
> He described a woman with a brain tumor that had characteristics of some other tumor that was not brain tumor-primary. He treats it not as though it's a brain tumor, but according to these other characteristics. It's working. It has nothing to do anymore with where it came from. He said, "Pathways create opportunities for treatments. It's like that's the nuts and bolts of it. That's the easy part—the basic science, the translational science."
>
> He talked more about precision medicine: "The more difficult thing is how it affects a person and how the mind is involved with that. The bigger challenge for me is how to

have my patients be happy and enjoy life, or if that's too ambitious, at least have life be valuable. Take cytokines for example. They're transmitters known to cause fever, fatigue, elevated white blood cell count. But 'good cytokines' can enhance dopamine release, feelings of well-being, etcetera. There are so many things which we don't understand, but will likely be tied together."

He said he, too, is curious about the mind-body interaction. He said,

"We can look at crude things like levels of cortisol and amino acid suppression. I think it's much more sophisticated. The geneticists have been surprised there aren't that many genes. There's a much higher homology between flies and humans. With epigenetics, what "things" are turned on? What makes these things work? It's subtle. What turns them on and off is much more environmental. You can turn on whether that gene gets used or not. But it's extremely personal—there are many ways you can combine things. That's the challenge. It's smart that people are coping with cancer, that we ought to keep working on our brains and understand things. What I know about life, and convince my patients, like you, is that we don't know what's going to happen to anybody. Especially somebody that has a certain kind of disease. Some diseases are predictable. Cancer is not predictable. Smokers' lung cancer used to be predictable. Sometimes there are genetic abnormalities; that just changes everything."

He described another patient:

"She got non-smokers' lung cancer. It was eating away at her bones. She didn't want to do anything. She tried to take her own life. We managed to get beyond that. We began to treat it in a targeted way—with medication to treat the epidermal growth factor which is relevant in some cancers. She started treatment; she takes some of these pills. It's been six years now. Her disease keeps shrinking, a little bit all the time. She comes in now every six to nine months and she's fine."

Epigenetics

Epigenetics is the study of changes in organisms as the result of modification of gene expression. It began in the middle of the twentieth century as research focused on combining genetics and developmental biology. The term epigenetics was coined in 1942 from the Greek word "epigenesis," which originally described how genetic processes affect development. In the nineteen-nineties, scientists studied in more detail "genetic assimilation"—that is, how an environmentally induced phenotype, or "acquired characteristic," becomes genetically fixed, such that the original stimulus that induced the change isn't needed anymore. Since then, research has focused on trying to understand the mechanisms for how these types of changes occur. We know of epigenetic modifications in DNA methylation, chromatin remodeling, histone modifications, and non-coding RNA mechanisms.

To translate: You might think of how this happens as Dr. Barstis hinted at—the common analogy is to think of gene expression like "switches" that get "turned on" or "turned off." The gene expression can be turned on and off by all sorts of factors, for example by a combination of lifestyle and environmental factors. These can be reflected at various times in a person's life. But it turns out, gene expression can also be affected by wars, famine, migration, slavery, genocide, trauma—essentially, by both personal and human history.

And such changes do not only affect the person who lives through them: Evidence shows that the descendants or third generation of the people who went through these experiences are affected, too. For example, human epidemiological studies show that prenatal and early postnatal environmental factors influence risk of these children, when they become adults, developing certain chronic diseases.[56] Dutch children born during what came to be called the Hunger Winter, the famine during 1944-1945 as a result of the Nazis occupying the Netherlands, show increased rates of obesity and coronary heart disease after their mothers lived through famine in early pregnancy, compared to those not exposed to famine. How do we explain this? Less DNA methylation of the IFG2 gene (insulin-like growth factor II), was found to be associated with the mothers who went through the famine during early pregnancy.[57]

This is fascinating to consider regarding cancer. The BRCA1 and 2 genetic mutations are "typographical errors" in tumor suppressor genes. They occur rarely in the general population, but among certain populations, the incidence is much higher. For example, Ashkenazi Jewish women are ten times as likely as the general population to have a BRCA1 or BRCA2 mutation.[58] There is a lot of conjecture about why certain populations have a higher rate of certain genetic mutations, but the general consensus is that, like all genetic change, if a group is isolated and does not intermarry, the genetic change persists and is passed down. Ashkenazi Jews historically did not intermarry, but instead married and had children within the small pool of their own shtetl communities.

From the perspective of energy healing, if we consider cells as having consciousness, if a "typo" began in someone's genes, why would that be passed down? Essentially, what this means cellularly is, if a cancer starts in someone with one of these mutations, the body's ability to suppress that tumor—through slowing down cell division, or repairing DNA mistakes, or programming the cancer cells to die—that ability is turned off in that person.

I am curious about the possible mind-body connection here. I am not a scientist, and I am aware that my question arises out of ignorance. I also understand that there is no survival advantage, so far as we know at the present time, for having one of the tumor suppressor genes like either of the BRCA genes. But, like Tolstoy, in the epigraph in our chapter on discernment, I want to pose the question here, in the hopes someone else will take it up and research further: Why would the consciousness of the cells essentially say "Don't stop! Make more cells." I can imagine, far too easily I'm afraid, what it might feel like to go through a pogrom. Sometimes I feel, in my body, a visceral fear, a sense of easily being able to kinesthetically feel (or remember?) what it is like to be that afraid. You're in your house. It is nighttime. You are trying to hide. There is nowhere to hide, really. You know the Cossacks are coming to your shtetl. You know that doesn't go well. You're trying to be as still as possible, so quiet your breathing will not be apparent. Hopefully, they won't come. But you know they will. They will break down the door, shatter all the dishes, slit open the feather pillows, kill all the men (your husband, your father, your grandfather, your brothers).

They may rape you and/or kill you and all the women (your sister, your mother, your daughter).

If you survive and there's a belief system that you are hated, other, foreign, somehow both Chosen, and bad, can you imagine how you might misunderstand, get confused, and feel, from this belief system, "I don't want to die. I'm not bad. I'm afraid. We're hated. We are being killed. We must make more of us. Make more! Make more cells!"

I realize how preposterous and unscientific this both sounds and is. And yet, this kinesthetic experience has been a part of how I feel, in my body, for as long as I can remember. Until hearing of this field of epigenetics, I never mentioned it to anyone. Now I find I'm curious: What's it like to live that way my whole life? What effect does this have on my cells? Where did I even get this idea, growing up in then safe America? Why is it so familiar to me in my body, so specific that I can see the wooden breakfront that holds the dishes, the pattern of red and yellow flowers on the borders of the plates and bowls? I know the layout of the small house. I know where each piece of furniture is and what it looks like, how it feels to brush my hands against the solid wood of the table, how it feels to sleep on a scratchy mattress on the bed (does it have straw inside?) there with my body. When I'm in this experience, I can feel my breathing gets shallow—now, in my body today—my muscle tension and the surface tension on my skin increases. I did not live through any pogrom. But my ancestors did. It must have been bad; it was severe enough that my great-grandfather walked from Berdichev in what's now the Ukraine—he walked to Italy (!) (that's more than two-thousand kilometers, more than thirteen-hundred miles). He worked there to bring in the grape harvest, for two years, apparently. Then he made his way to Rotterdam, where he sailed to Canada. Eventually, he saved money and brought over his family, one by one. They did not know how to farm, and so moved to Detroit, Michigan, when Henry Ford was offering five dollars a day to work in the car factories. A notorious anti-Semite, Ford refused to hire any Jews. My family did not work in the Ford Motor plant, but instead some worked construction, others (on my maternal grandmother's side) started a market. After several years, all the brothers on my paternal grandfather's side (the side with the BRCA1 gene), had saved enough money to send one of them to college. They chose my grandfather, and he became a dentist. (We think he likely had the BRCA1 gene, as he died of esophageal/stomach cancer at age seventy. He likely passed it on to my mother, who passed it on to me.)

I wish I could say this experience (or memory?) is just evidence of me having a vivid imagination or being some "strange" healer who invents "things." But it turns out there is research supporting the idea that we carry memories of experiences we never personally lived through, but that our ancestors did. Anne Ancelin Schutzenberger, a child psychologist in France, has written a book which details her observation of this phenomenon in many children in her private practice. In *The Ancestor Syndrome: Transgenerational Psychotherapy and the Hidden Links in the Family Tree,*[59] Schutzenberger describes all kinds of physical and emotional symptoms that make concerned parents bring their kids to see her. For example, one child had severe asthma. He'd typically have a nightmare and wake in the midst of having an asthma attack. He was very young, if I remember correctly, age three or so, far too young to have an abstract understanding of psychology. She asked him to draw what he dreamt that frightened him. He drew an army helmet with a point on top. These helmets, it turned out, corresponded to helmets worn by the German infantry during the Battle of Verdun in the First World War. It turned out that his relative, I believe it was his grandfather, had fought at Verdun, which marked the first time in history that mustard gas was used. His grandfather had been there. Some of the soldiers had functional gas masks; others were exposed and died horribly painful deaths. When inhaled, mustard gas causes bleeding and blistering within the respiratory system; people die two days later. Schutzenberger became curious if this little boy was having a "memory" of the Battle of Verdun, long before his lifetime, but where his grandfather fought. The asthma in him today would have been the response to not being able to breathe as the mustard gas burned the soldiers' respiratory systems.

Mind-Body Attempts to Influence Gene Expression and Health

Schutzenberger studies emotional issues. Researchers in the US have studied children born to mothers who were pregnant and lived near Ground Zero in New York City on September 11, 2001. Some seventeen hundred women who were pregnant on 9/11 lived near Ground Zero or were in the World Trade Center towers. The women who were in their third trimester of pregnancy who subsequently were diagnosed with PTSD showed low levels of cortisol in their saliva a year later. So did their babies.[60] In other words, their mothers' experience somehow predisposed the babies to PTSD. Babies of women who were pregnant on 9/11 and lived near Ground Zero also were small for their gestational age, and they experienced developmental delays.[61]

I am curious how much of what our ancestors went through may be affecting the generations alive today. Is the increasing rate of cancer in the West today in any way connected to experiences our ancestors went through? What effects might the events of today have on future generations of our offspring? If there are shown to be any effects, knowing that, can we affect epigenetic gene expression by being aware of it and offering some remediation to deal with the issues? This question takes us back to the mind-body connection questions at the beginning of the book. The notion that we might be able to affect our health favorably—in general, not just in terms of gene expression—through mind-body connection, is one of the main areas of exploration of this whole book.

The Medicine of the Future

At the beginning of the book, in the Introduction, I called for more research to see if the Thriving Through Cancer Method has any effect on overall survival, progression-free survival, or "merely" quality of life. I am not alone in wanting to have increased dialogue between conventional, allopathic medicine and complementary, integrative healing modalities. I dream of a world in which we compare notes, share best practices, and use everything that works. Dr. Friedman articulated that desire this way:

> "I'd like to see a study that systematically looks at complementary medicine in oncology patients. That study does not exist. In the future, we're going to see clinical trials studying the utility of complementary medicine. I want to see an active clinical trial program. I'd like to know what the answer is myself. If complementary medicine is shown to improve quality of life and survival, then everybody should be getting it; it shouldn't be self-selected. If it's not working, then people shouldn't waste their time and money."[62]

Dr. Chrysopoulo, one of the early surgeons to perform the Alloderm All-in-One breast reconstruction surgery puts it this way:

"We're still in a time of dialogue being somewhat new. There's still a lot of ignorance." I shared with him my story of the supplements prescribed by my functional MD that interacted with the chemo. And how I was shocked that there was no dialogue between the functional MD and the hematologist-oncologist. He was already familiar with my experience of my local breast surgeons being angry and saying awfully condescending remarks that I'd travel to have a different doctor perform the breast surgery in a new way. Dr. Chrysopoulo said,

> "The default position right now is one of antagonism, for example of one doctor towards another. Someone comes and passes on information from another physician. The default is to raise your eyebrow rather than listening to what the patient is saying. Okay. You think to yourself: The doctor said this? You're listening to the interpretation of the patient, who has no medical background. There's no need to put the doctor down to the patient. We hear about it from our out of state patients. The local physician didn't want the patient to travel. They say to the patient [about the new way he and the other surgeons in his practice do breast reconstructions] 'They're not special. If you stay here, it may not be the same procedure, but it will be just as good.'"

It's not just doctors who employ different surgical techniques however, where we need more open dialogue. In this day and age, where records can be electronically transmitted and email makes communication virtually instantaneous, we can have greater communication if we simply set up systems (i.e., enough time scheduled in a clinical day) to foster it. When I was facing the "big surgery," of the incision all the way up "the length of me" (from my pubic bone all the way to my xiphoid), I knew I was facing also the surgical placing of a Port-a-Cath to receive chemo. The question arose of whether I should have one port or two. Dr. Friedman was certain that based on my high CA-125, he'd find a lot of cancer, so he wanted me to get two ports—one an intraperitoneal (or IP) one in my pelvis, and the other one near my collarbone that would have a tube that runs into my subclavian vein and from there into my heart. The advantage to having the IP port, too, would be some chemo could go through the port into my pelvis, and essentially dump the chemo right there, near where my fallopian tubes used to be, and where the cancer had originated. By the upper port putting chemo directly into my heart, it would immediately get pumped throughout my bloodstream.

Dr. Barstis wanted me to only get the port to my heart—he wanted the widespread distribution of chemo to every part of my body. Dr. Friedman knows survival is maximized when chemo is concentrated where the cancer is. Dr. Barstis argued that I had had a recurrence near my mediastinum, far from my pelvis, so we really needed chemo not concentrated but spread throughout my body.

Because Dr. Friedman and Dr. Barstis are at two different institutions, and because those two were at that time not on the same network, so not able to share big electronic files such as imaging studies, it was not so easy for them to confer. In the week when I had said yes to surgery and it was scheduled, but the two doctors hadn't yet managed to reach each other, I had an emotional meltdown with James. Busy clinical days don't really allow time for such phone calls between doctors easily. It was not James' fault, but I became sad and furious: "It's Friday, and my surgery is Tuesday. I'm afraid I'll be 'under' on the table, they won't have reached each other, and you won't know how to communicate to them what I want!" So patiently, James said, "Okay. Start again. Explain all this to me and tell me what you want." The man is a saint. I said, "I don't want two ports unless we're going to use them both. If we're not going to use the one in my pelvis, I don't want it. Please tell them if I can't." He said he would.

That night, on a Friday night at eleven p.m., I got an email from Dr. Barstis. "We finally talked. We agree. One port unless there are three or more lesions. If more than that, then two." He reiterated that he likes Dr. Friedman and trusts him. I calmed down.

But it shouldn't be this way. Doctors work so hard. We have the technology that consultations like this can be potentially very easy—a simple, secure email. The HIPAA law in the US, meant to preserve patient confidentiality so no one is discriminated against for health information, has as a consequence this slowing down of communication. It's time to revisit how we can set up a system that preserves patients' rights, and yet fosters sharing of relevant medical information, such as imaging studies and charts. We need more dialogue; we need more conversation. We would collectively benefit from care being routinely multidisciplinary.

Once again, I'm struck by the different style of medical care in the Netherlands. My doctors there meet in a weekly multidisciplinary panel to discuss patients' cases and recommendations for the best care. After they meet, their recommendations are posted on my chart that I can access via the hospital's secure website. That site is, of course, password protected. But it also involves a double layer of security. As I log in, I click a link that sends a request to my Digital ID, a digital identification system in the Netherlands. Once my login is electronically deemed to be legitimate (from one of my devices) I then receive a text message with a unique code on my mobile phone. The code is different every time I log in. I enter that uniquely-generated code along with my username and password, and I can read the panel's recommendations. I can also see my chart, including imaging, reports, blood work, treatments, next appointments, etcetera. I know I'll see my doctor soon, and we can discuss the recommendations. I also know that part of her day is devoted to calling patients. If needed, I can call the main number of the hospital, and they can look up for me approximately what time she'll call me. If I happen to need to call her, and it's after the workday, unless it's an emergency, the assistant on duty will usually say something like, "Can it wait until tomorrow?" So far, I've only needed to call after-hours once. And when asked, I realized my issue could wait. I respect the time boundaries of the Dutch in so many areas of life. When they work, they work. When they're not at work, they completely stop working and live life. This returns sanity to everyone, including doctors, nurses, and patients alike.

I'd also like to see medical literacy taught, just like other skills in life. The British chef Jamie Oliver has taught "food literacy," the planning, selection, preparation and eating of food. Eating is obviously needed for survival, but many of us do not know anymore how to cook. Oliver set out to teach these skills. Medical literacy strikes me as similar. Whether we have a life-threatening illness or not, we all, throughout our lives, need to know basic skills about medicine and healthcare. Right now, those skills are not common knowledge, and they are not taught. The situation my "California Mom" went through, with the staph infection in her arm, the same bacteria that meant my parents' friend lost his life, the friend that had malaria, but he didn't know to mention he had lived in India a year prior, and the attending didn't know to ask—these kinds of situations wouldn't happen if we all knew what to look for and how to communicate what we observe. The trend of patient-as-consumer that started in the nineties can now, if we choose, expand into greater knowledge on the part of patients, and knowledge of how to communicate with healthcare professionals at initial intake to improve care.

It is my dream that this Thriving Through Cancer Method can contribute to the necessary integration between medicine and healing, between large medical bodies of health insurance companies, hospitals, and governmental organizations—with our personal, individual bodies, yours and mine.

It is my intention that this Method can serve as a bridge—so you can come to know yourself well, moment by moment, you can perceive and communicate your needs, and you can use practices like those presented here—to live your life filled both with the sense of your own vitality and wonder at the presence of all life.

APPENDIX

--

WORKSHEETS

Worksheet 1
from Breadcrumbs on the Path Home:
Your Personal Life Experience

Your Personal Life Experience

This worksheet accompanies The Need for the TTC Method from a Personal Perspective chapter.

1. What was your childhood like? What was valued in your family?
   A. Physical
   B. Emotional
   C. Mental
   D. Spiritual

2. How did that show up in how you spent time as a child/which activities did you enjoy? Which did you pursue? (e.g., reading, sports, music, dance, religious school, scouts, debate, crafts, art, science club, etcetera).

3. Was one set of skills valued to exclusion of other skills (e.g., reading/intellectual prowess over dancing/any physical activity?)

4. What about during your teenage years—what did you love to do? What piqued your curiosity? Were you permitted/encouraged or discouraged/punished for spending time and energy on what naturally drew you?

5. What about as a young adult—how did you choose what to do for work? Was there any expectation that you should fulfill certain role(s)?

    A. If so, what were these role(s)?

    B. Did you fulfill these joyfully, because they naturally fit what you were interested in, or did you comply, and squeeze yourself into work/role based on expectations from someone outside of yourself (for example your family, your education, your class)?

6. What about now? Where are you now with these issues? Do your choices fit you? Do you have any regrets in life? If so, what are they, especially around these issues?

WORKSHEET 2
QUALITIES IMPORTANT TO YOU
AS A PRACTITIONER AND/OR PATIENT

This worksheet accompanies the How I Became an Energy Healer chapter.

Whether you're the healthcare practitioner or the patient (or both), it's useful to consider what qualities you bring and what qualities you look for in each role.

For example, if you're a patient going through cancer, what qualities do you want your doctors to possess? Do you want different qualities in different doctors? For example, do you want your surgeon to have certain qualities and your oncologist to meet different needs, and so to have different qualities? For example, you might prefer a surgeon who'll be very thorough and will work on you in the O.R. "like a car mechanic, tinkering away under the hood," (in your body), for hours, to get every last shred of cancer out. This surgeon might not have a "warm and fuzzy" bedside manner, but maybe that's okay with you if you can get that need met elsewhere, such as in your oncologist, if you have that need.

Also, as the patient, what qualities do you want to bring to your appointments? Do you want to know a lot or not know anything, and just have the doctors "decide what to do"? Or somewhere in the middle? You actually have a lot of choice in how you experience going through the disease and treatment process. At the very least, you get to choose your doctor, the hospital where you're treated, the culture and environment of the place, and what else, if anything, you want to do.

If you're the practitioner, you, too, can use this worksheet. As the practitioner, what qualities do you bring to your patients? What makes you unique? Why would particular patients choose to work with you specifically? Trust these qualities are your strengths.

As the practitioner, what kinds of patients do you most enjoy working with? What qualities in patients makes your work most rewarding? Knowing these qualities, can you "train your patients," so they know what you like? For example, you might assign your patient time to think about a potential treatment—for example, to see if she's willing to try a certain chemo drug, while you consider the possibilities. You can ask her to think about it and let you know what she wants at your next appointment. Do you prefer your patients to email you or not, but rather to email or call your staff? You often get to choose these details in your practice.

Patients, you, too, can "train" your doctors by asking them directly, "Do you prefer I email you, or just be in contact with your assistant? Do you suggest I read/review/or learn anything to help us decide if this is the preferred method of treatment now?"

So now, both patients and practitioners, turn your attention to the list of qualities below, as well as any other qualities you can think of. You can choose as many or as few qualities as you want. Rank these qualities according to three categories:

1. Necessary;
2. Would like to have/be;
3. Would be nice.

Rank the qualities you choose under each category. Then fill in the qualities you want in your practitioner and in yourself and write those qualities, in order, under each area. If you want to get fancy, you can assign percentage points to the qualities/categories, as in, "This quality is seventy-five percent important to me. This one is only five percent." If you do this, make sure you end up with one hundred percent.

Here are the qualities:

Tenacious
Intelligent
Proactive
Curious
Tolerant

Open-minded

Open to alternatives

Willing to discuss

Generous with time, attention

Good at observing

Good at personalizing/tailoring treatment protocol to you

Holistic

Embodied

Communicative

Steady

Reassuring

Warm

Personable

No nonsense

Up to date on latest techniques/research

Leader in field

Pioneering

Willing to share success rates

Willing to share pictures (of surgical results)

Experienced

Published

Articulate

Respected by colleagues

Respected by other patients

Positive reviews

Member of appropriate governing board

Part of teaching hospital

Not part of teaching hospital

Admitting privileges at hospital/center you like

Looks and sounds like they take good care of themselves

Healthy

Happy

Good boundaries

Not getting needs met by patients-healthy relationships outside of practice

Good eye contact

Access to excellent resources

Happy support staff

Pleasant environment

Accessible

Concerned with your quality of life

Respectful

Timely

Punctual

Present

Good systems

Organized

Remembers details about you, your situation, your preferences, your care

Attentive

Reveals the amount of information you want

Emotional

Dispassionate

Factual

Hopeful

Willing to connect you/refer you to others

Creative

Engaged with practice

Smart

Bright

Asks good questions

Good listener

Follows treatment recommendations

Tweaks treatment recommendations

Shares openly

Good at brainstorming

Integrative

Compliant

Responsible

Loyal

Deeply-feeling

Responsive

Willing

Trusting

Trustworthy

Determined

Ally

Partner

In touch with emotions

As you consider the list, now rank, in order, which qualities you feel are necessary, which qualities would you like to have, and which would be nice. You can choose as many or few qualities as you want in each category.

If you complete this worksheet and realize your current practitioner is not meeting your needs, this clearly allows you to switch and find someone who does. As you "shop around," for your right practitioners, having your list, you'll be able to quickly and easily choose who is right for you.

If you're the patient, and you realize you'd like to transform your experience, you can do that right away, or ask yourself what you need in order to feel and behave differently.

If you're the practitioner, the same applies but in reverse: what qualities do you want to bring as the practitioner? Rank these in order of, Necessary, Would Like to Be/Have, Would Be Nice.

The same goes if you're the practitioner completing the worksheet for the types of patients you most enjoy working with. What qualities are necessary to allow you to enjoy working with that patient? Which qualities would you like to see? Which would be nice? Rank these in order. You can have as many or as few qualities as you wish. If you wish, you can assign percentages to each quality/set of qualities. Make sure your total adds up to 100 percent.

Qualities in a Practitioner

Necessary:

_____

_____

_____

_____

Would like to have/be:

_____

_____

_____

_____

Would be nice:

_____

_____

_____

_____

Qualities as a Patient

Necessary:

_____

_____

_____

_____

Would like to have/be:

_____

_____

_____

_____

Would be nice:

_____

_____

_____

_____

WORKSHEET 3
YOUR BASELINE BEFORE
SELF-TRACKING

This worksheet accompanies the Self-Tracking and Tracking Others chapter.

The first step of the TTC Method is to take a baseline reading of where you are right now. This can be done sitting, standing or lying down. Just by paying attention to yourself right now, in this very moment, what do you notice:

Are you sitting? Standing? Lying down? _____

How's your breathing? Shallow, or deep? _____

Any areas of physical pain or tension? _____

If so, where? _____

What's it like? _____

How's your mood? _____

How are you feeling emotionally? _____

How's your mind? Any "chatter" going on? _____

Any awareness of how you're feeling spiritually?_____

Connected? _____

Not unified? _____

Anything else you notice? _____

There are no right or wrong answers, here. You're just observing. This is your baseline reading. As you do the first practice, Self-Tracking, you may notice that you feel different after.

*Also, this worksheet assumes you're filling in words. But feel free to adapt it in any way that suits you. Perhaps you'd rather draw a picture of what you sense or make note of any information using any of your senses, smell, for example. This is meant to be just a quick observation of where you are right now.

As you get good at this exercise, you can do it at any time—at work, on the subway, as you listen to someone or something.

WORKSHEET 4
SELF-TRACKING:
WHAT YOUR BODY REVEALS

1. Where in your body did you notice anything? Where were you drawn?

2. What did you notice?

3. What senses did you use? Did you
see/hear/smell/taste/touch/feel/experience/just know there? What was there?

4. Did more than one of your senses support you in what you sensed? For
example, did you see and just know? Or did you see and hear? Or was only
one sense involved (for example, did you feel, but not use any other senses to
confirm what you felt)?

5. Were you able to "be with" what you noticed, or did you want to change it somehow?

6. Did what you perceive connect to any situation currently going on in your life? Make a note of whatever you observed, even if you don't know how it's relevant yet.

7. If you didn't sense anything, did your body give you any answers/any clues about why not?

8. If so, what were those answers or clues?

9. Can you give yourself what your body gave you answers/clues about that you need?

10. If not now, can you get clear on when you can give yourself what your body is letting you know you need?

11. If yes, can you schedule that now?

12. If your body is not giving you any clues or answers as to what you need, did you ask your body why not? Did you sense any reply?

13. If you did sense a reply, what did you perceive? It might be literal, and it might be symbolic (for example, a picture, or a sound, a smell, etcetera). Any way you perceive is fine.

14. What sense(s) did you use?

15. Can you now give yourself what your body let you know you need, in order to have the dialogue or conversation about your deeper needs/wants?

16. If so, when/how can you give that to yourself?

17. If not, why not?

18. How does your body feel about that?

19. How is this experience for you? Would you like to adjust it in some way so that it works for you? If so, how? You can do that now.

WORKSHEET 5
ASSESSMENT TO FOSTER DISCERNMENT

This worksheet accompanies the Assessment to Foster Discernment chapter.

Just like the first step of the TTC Method is to take a baseline reading of where you are right now, so, too, you take a baseline often. Here we'll do it before and after the stories that accompany the tool Assessment to Foster Discernment. This worksheet is in two parts. The first part, the Baseline, is a copy of what you filled out before the first tool, Self-Tracking. The second part of the worksheet tracks what shifts as you read the stories connected with that tool.

Baseline:

This can be done sitting, standing or lying down. Just by paying attention to yourself right now, in this very moment, what do you notice:

Are you sitting? Standing? Lying down? _____

How's your breathing? Shallow, or deep? _____

Any areas of physical pain or tension? _____

If so, where? _____

What's it like? _____

How's your mood? _____

How are you feeling emotionally? _____

How's your mind? Any "chatter" going on? _____

Any awareness of how you're feeling spiritually? _____

Connected? _____

Not unified? _____

Anything else you notice? _____

There are no right or wrong answers, here. You're just observing. This is your baseline reading. As you do the first practice, Self-Tracking, you may notice that you feel different after.

*Also, this worksheet assumes you're filling in words. But feel free to adapt it in any way that suits you. Perhaps you'd rather draw a picture of what you sense or make note of any information using any of your senses, smell, for example. This is meant to be just a quick observation of where you are right now.

As you get good at this exercise, you can do it at any time—at work, in transit, as you listen to someone else.

After reading the stories in Assessment to Foster Discernment:

Notice if these stories evoke any feelings in you. How do you feel?

Angry? _____

Sad? _____

Confident? _____

Doubtful? _____

What happens to your breathing as you read the stories in Assessment to Foster Discernment?

_____

_____

Do you notice any shifts that happen in your body? If so, what do you notice specifically (for example, what happens to any areas of tension, for example, does your stomach tighten as you read these stories?

_____

_____

Can you observe what happens, what gets evoked in you with no demand that you change anything arising in you? What happens in you?

_____

_____

_____

WORKSHEET 6
PUTTING TOGETHER YOUR PRACTICES

This worksheet accompanies the Putting Together Your Practices chapter.

Here make note of any needs you noticed as you worked the four tools of the Assessment. What needs do you have right now in any and every level—physically, emotionally, mentally and spiritually?

Physical

Emotional

Mental

Spiritual

WORKSHEET 7
YOUR MENU OF PRACTICES

This worksheet is part of the Physical, Emotional, Mental and Spiritual Practices chapters.

Refer to your worksheet "Putting Together Your Practices," where you noted your needs in every area of your life. Now fill in which practices you sense will help you meet the needs you identified on that worksheet. Keep in mind that the practices are synergistic, that is, as you work each area, your whole life develops more than if you only work with one area at a time.

The practices in the method are meant to be a jumping off point. If you'd like, feel free to generate your own practices to meet your needs. Write those down here, too. After you have them all written down, decide when you want to work each one. You can commit as much or as little time as you wish. You get to choose. As you get familiar with using the method, you'll be able to ascertain at any given time which practice or set of practices is called for at any moment, to meet any of your needs.

Physical

Emotional

Mental

Spiritual

When Do You Plan to Work Each One?

_____
_____
_____
_____
_____
_____
_____

Acknowledgments

When I first said out loud in 2010 that I was developing a method of mind-body integration for health and that I was going to write this book, my idea was to synthesize everything I knew from my training in energy healing with what I learned in my years of dancing, choreographing, performing and studying theatre. I felt shy, because while I knew I love to live this way, my intellectual education and upbringing discounted these holistic, integrative, embodied ways of knowing, and I always privileged the intellectual and rational above these other modes of perception.

Being diagnosed with cancer in 2012 changed that. I now saw there was "no time like the present," and further, that the Assessment tools and Practices were helping me have a very different experience going through cancer than that of other people I knew who also were sick with various types of cancer. Several of those friends have since died. I miss them. I don't know if this material has helped me stay alive, but it has not harmed me. And given my prognosis, I'm happy to be here.

I realized this material may be useful to others besides me.

Yet while a labor of love, sometimes this book felt like a project of desperation: those were the times I did not trust that I'd live long enough to finish it. Yet working with these Practices, I actually felt well most of the time.

There are countless people to thank. My husband James supported me in all ways big and small—these are just some of the ways he shows his love: James listened to my ideas, writing style, ways of structuring and teaching. He cooked me innumerable meals, and designed the cover of this book. Even more than these tangible demonstrations, he supported me emotionally at every turn, in all kinds of intangible ways, through the full range of moods—when I was sad or exhausted during grueling treatments as well as when I was brimming with ideas, excited about the work. His love and patience helped birth this book. My mother, Nancy Klein, brought her incisive questions, her brilliant mind and background in philosophy to help me ground the perspectives expressed here in the history of ideas. Jerry Klein always let me know by his questions that he's curious and wants to know more, even when going through his own health challenges—that's a wisdom I admire. My sister, Barbara Hahn, PhD, author of two books with the third one close to completion, taught me the law of diminishing returns—that is, how to write as well as possible, and get the book done. My Uncle Bill and Aunt Ricki Cohen always asked how the writing was coming, and I could tell by their frequent phone calls and the little catch in their voices when they asked about my health every time, that they love me, want me to live, and support any project I put my mind to. James' parents, my "California Mom and Dad," John and Dee Ann Roche, loved me steadily throughout my fears and seemingly endless rounds of chemo. They'd coax me out of my office lair with offers of conversation and they'd ply me with brunch. Dad even spent hours changing my cold caps once, so I wouldn't lose my hair from the chemo. Thank you. My brother and sister-in-law, Mike and Gina Roche, and kids Deon and Jackie, were a warm family presence. Teri Abbott made delicious soups, shared wonderful conversation, her blooming plants, peaceful home, and her own mind-body-spirit way of listening and sharing, as well as her passion for alternative medicine.

This book would literally not have been possible without my doctors, nurses, and healers. They are my heroes, and words cannot convey how grateful I am that they have helped me stay alive. John Barstis, MD strategized my case so creatively—he accomplished the goal of keeping me "alive and strong" so I could (if I need it in the future) take advantage of all the medications (and perhaps other treatments) that are coming down the pipeline. He is a great listener, and so supportive of each new, grand project—whether that meant teaching in Massachusetts, traveling for months at a time, and then immigrating to the Netherlands. The nurses at UCLA— Angie Alejo, Elaine Colangelo, Michelle Gorman, Siobhan Davis—provided warmth, care, soothing ways of helping me get through the sixteen months of chemotherapy there. The whole UCLA team—Cynthia Carsten, Kimberlee Torp, Veronica Magana, Ryan Gayon, Elvia Lopez, Sarah Fitzgerald, Katie Orefice, Mayra Saucedo, Roxana Gonzalez, Donna Ashmore, Manjeet Wahi and Mindy Burgess—together create an office where patients can relax and trust, because they handle all the details of our care so well. Joan MacIntosh launched me into exploring the world of energy healing and supported me getting my creativity back. Irene Tobler demonstrated by personal example teachings on mindfulness and how to be present.

Richard Friedman, MD also saved my life. His qualities of open-heartedness, brilliance, and tenacity in the OR have kept hundreds, if not thousands, of women alive. That makes his job harder, as his waiting room fills with more of us survivors who need check-ups, but we are forever grateful to him. I loved our conversations. Helen Zadourian, RN, BSN, OCN, always communicated all the details back and forth, and made me feel she truly cared that I live. Zhanna provided righteous anger that also likely saved my life when she said, "If it were me, I'd get in here right away! Do not wait two weeks!" Roxanne and Christy kept everything humming smoothly.

Minas Chrysopoulo, MD is a pioneer in new surgical techniques that help those of us fortunate enough to be his patients to keep our dignity and sense of ourselves in our bodies. He is a mensch, a great human being. His ability to put himself in the shoes of his patients is an exceptional gift. Denise Campos "holds" all of Dr. Chrysopoulo's patients so well, with a lightheartedness that helps us relax.

Dr. Carolien Smorenburg is an exceptional doctor. She inherited my huge case, learned and remembered all the details, and always asks just the right questions. I trust her, and admire her for how she cares for her patients with authenticity and discernment. Dr. Wouter Vogel taught me the benefits of radiotherapy and designed and oversaw my treatment. Based on his recommendations, I went from thinking I did not want radiation, to feeling I did. And he set it up in such a way that I could keep writing and still teach in the States. Kiki Firch is always warm, helpful, and willing to teach me the details how healthcare works here in the Netherlands. The many nurses and radiotherapy techs I've met at the Antoni van Leeuwenhoek hospital in Amsterdam have my supreme gratitude.   And they've taught me a little Dutch as they've treated me.

In Miami, Martha Pereira, ARNP: Her humor, attentiveness and brilliance were so helpful at the beginning stages back in 2012. I'm still alive, and since we're no longer in Florida, she is missed. Jeanette Lewis, RN, amazingly, kept us all correctly hooked up to our pumps, with grace and fortitude, through the thick of her solo twelve-hour workdays.

Thank you to Pedro Ramirez, MD, MD Anderson, and Jack Watkins, formerly there.

Thank you to the doctors I interviewed for this book. Steve Cole, PhD—Before we lived in Los Angeles, I heard and watched some of his lectures at UCLA via YouTube. When James and I moved to LA, and so Steve and I met in person a couple of years later, and I asked my preliminary question: "If perceived social isolation affects gene expression in metastasis and recurrence of ovarian cancer, are we at the stage yet when a doctor could prescribe to the woman in that situation, 'Get new friends'?" he answered, "You waited two years? You would've thought you'd send an email or something." Our conversation that followed and his research informs this whole book—he has deepened my understanding of the interaction of emotions and gene expression. He has also convinced me that my eudaimonic joy in writing may very well be helping me live long and well.

Arash Asher, MD, is emotionally sensitive, kinesthetically perceptive, and willing to talk about the emotional and spiritual needs of people going through advanced disease.

Many people coaxed and nurtured this book at every stage. Rasmani Deborah Orth, EdD, senior programmer at Kripalu, has been both patient and curious: Each year when I'd return to teach energy healing there, she'd say about this work in her lovely drawl, "Oooh—that sounds really fascinating. We'd love to have you teach it here. Keep me posted when you're ready." Lisa Anselme, Executive Director of Healing Beyond Borders, the organization of nurses certified in Healing Touch, invited me to give the keynote at the annual conference in 2015 that marked the first public presentation of this work. The several hundred nurses who heard it and earned continuing education credits for this material let me know I was on the right track. Martha Williams at 1440 Multiversity has graciously and warmly invited me to teach this work at the new center in California. Chris Bledy wrote the book, *Beating Ovarian Cancer*, which led me to both Dr. Barstis and Dr. Friedman.

Many people helped by reviewing drafts, and discussing methods for writing. Loolwa Khazzoom gave feedback on early and more recent drafts. Izabella and Michael Wentz taught me so much about getting a book written, published, and successfully distributed. If they still lived in Amsterdam we'd have more long conversations with Boomer on my lap. Shelli Stanger Nelson: my fellow healer friend, fellow teacher and writer has woven in and through my life at key moments. Achim Nowak shared his inspiring experiences right when I needed to hear them over the past twenty-two years, and modeled for me how to make the final drafts complete.

Besides my family, several people have helped me create this amazing life: Jessica Turnoff Ferrari is always there, across the miles, and through the years. Michael Mervosh has spent years working with me—through my happiness, sadness, all the ups and downs of ordinary, heroic life. I am grateful for how he listens with his whole body and energy field. He fosters passionate aliveness in me, and in everyone around him. Yvet van Geest is a great friend, and she has generously helped us with every detail of immigration, from picking us up at Schiphol countless times at ungodly hours to answering all our questions over several years, to helping each of us brainstorm each new stage of James' business and my practice. Marijke Hajunga has welcomed us into her life. Gloria Stewart's instruction in MELT Method has given me back a sense of joy at being alive in my physical, human, vulnerable body. Dyana Valentine always remembers the details of surgery anniversaries, treatment dates, and cheered both me and this book on at every stage. I miss our brunches and lunches all over LA. Tamara Cheyette-Cohen, Naomi Coodin, and Amalour Veloso: Each live on in this work; zichronah livracha, for each of you—may your memories be for a blessing.

ABOUT THE AUTHOR

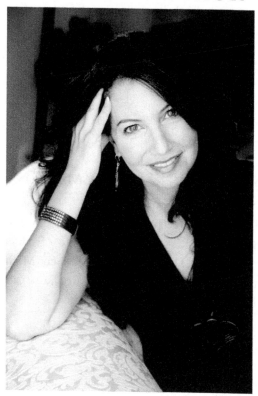

M elanie Roche is an energy healer and creator of the Thriving Through Cancer Method. A cancer survivor herself, she brings a wealth of experience in mind-body healing, meditation, therapy, dance, and theatre to lead personalized programs for thought leaders, patients, doctors, nurses, psychotherapists, and healers in all modalities. She served on the faculty at the Barbara Brennan School of Healing in Miami and Tokyo, working directly with Barbara Brennan. Melanie was invited—along with a physician and other holistic practitioners—to inaugurate the Integrative Health and Wellness Program at Canyon Ranch Miami Beach, the premier mind-body health resort, which attracts guests seeking a healthy lifestyle through comprehensive integration between medicine and healing. She coordinated an after-school program for high school students who plan to become physicians at New York University School of Medicine. In addition to her serving on the faculty and her eight years of training at the Barbara Brennan School of Healing, she also holds a BA in comparative religion from Columbia University and an MA in experimental theatre from New York University. Melanie leads workshops and speaks internationally. She lives in Amsterdam with her husband, James Roche.

http://www.MelanieRoche.com

WEBSITE/WORKSHOPS/MAILING LIST

Thank you for reading this book.

Join our mailing list and be part of the conversation and movement for integrative health. Get updates on the full range of Melanie's workshops, trainings, certification in the Thriving Through Cancer Method, new releases, bonus content, and other offerings by Melanie Roche. Visit online to sign up at: http://www.MelanieRoche.com.

ENDNOTES

[1] "What You Need to Know About 4 Gynecological Cancers." 2 June 2015, 16 Jul 2016. https://health.clevelandclinic.org/2015/06/what-you-need-to-know-about-4-gynecological-cancers/

[2] Early adoption of BRCA1/2 testing: who and why. Katrina Armstrong, Janet Weiner, Barbara Weber and David A Asch, Genetics in Medicine (2003) 5, 92-98 10 Jul. 2016.
http://www.ncbi.nlm.nih.gov/pubmed/12644778.

[3] The Role of Secondary Surgery in Recurrent Ovarian Cancer, D. Lorusso, M. Mancini, R. Di Rocco, R. Fontanelli, and F. Raspagliesi, Introduction International Journal of Surgical Oncology Volume 2012 (2012), Article ID 613980 Received 31 March 2012; Accepted 30 May 2012 10 Jul. 2016.
http://www.hindawi.com/journals/ijso/2012/613980/.

[4] For example, in the general population, the risk of having the BRCA1 or BRCA2 gene is 0.2 to 0.3 percent. "About BRCA1, BRCA2, and Hereditary Breast and Ovarian Cancers."
https://www.knowbrca.org/Provider/FNA/about-brca1-brca2-and-hereditary-breast-and-ovarian-cancers 16 Jul. 2016.
https://www.knowbrca.org/Provider/FNA/about-brca1-brca2-and-hereditary-breast-and-ovarian-cancers.

[5] Primary Carcinoma of the Fallopian Tube: Report of Two Cases with Literature Review, Cancer Res Treat. 2009 Jun; 41(2): 113–116.
Published online 30 June 2009 doi: 10.4143/crt.2009.41.2.113 PMCID: PMC2731206 21 Sept 2016
.http://www.ncbi.nlm.nih.gov/pmc/articles/PMC2731206/.

[6] Stage IV Ovarian Cancer. CancerConnect News. 23 Mar. 2004 21 Sept 2016.
http://news.cancerconnect.com/stage-iv-ovarian-cancer/.

[7] Personal interview with Minas Chrysopoulo, MD 26 May 2015.

[8] Crossing Brooklyn Ferry. (Leaves of Grass (1860-61)) - The Walt Whitman Archive. 23 Sep. 2016.
http://www.whitmanarchive.org/published/LG/1860/poems/122

[9] The History of the Internet in a Nutshell 15 Nov. 2009 24 Sep. 2016 http://sixrevisions.com/resources/the-history-of-the-internet-in-a-nutshell.

[10] The Barbara Brennan School of Healing collects research on the effects of Brennan Healing Science. Please contact the School via barbarabrennan.com for research papers.

[11] Body psychotherapy 22 May 2016 24 Sep. 2016.
https://en.wikipedia.org/w/index.php?title=Body_psychotherapy&oldid=721507414.

[12] See Alexander Lowen, The Language of the Body (1971), Stephen M Johnson, Character Styles (1994), and Barbara Brennan, Hands of Light (1988).

[13] Healing Beyond Borders Annual Conference 2015. I gave the keynote on 3 Oct 2015 on "The Joy of Presence: Why and How to Use Inner Directed Energy Awareness to Heal Ourselves, Patients and the World." (Inner Directed Energy Awareness, or The IDEA Method, is an application of this Method I developed for more general applications, not specifically for cancer.)

[14] Personal interview with John Barstis, MD 26 Mar. 2015.

[15] Susan Aposhyan, Susan. Body-Mind Psychotherapy: Principles, Techniques, and Practical Applications, Norton, 2004, p. 190.

[16] Personal interview with Arash Asher, MD. 23 June 2015.

[17] Personal interview with Steve Cole, PhD. 16 March 2015.

[18] Windelband, Wilhelm. History of Philosophy, revised ed f 1901. Harper & Bros f Harper Torchbooks 1958, pp. 404-406.
https://archive.org/stream/historyofphiloso02wind#page/406/mode/2up/search/spati-ality.Windelband 1958.

[19] René Descartes - Wikipedia.
https://en.wikipedia.org/wiki/Ren%C3%A9_Descartes. Accessed 16 Oct. 2016.

[20] Life Over Cancer: The Block Center Program for Integrative Cancer Treatment: Keith Block, Andrew Weil M.D.: 9780553801149: Amazon.com: Books. 16 Oct. 2016 https://www.amazon.com/Life-Over-Cancer-Integrative-
Treatment/dp/0553801147/ref=sr_1_1?ie=UTF8&qid=1476656537&sr=8-1&keywords=Block+cancer.

[21] Personal interview with Arash Asher, MD 23 June 2015.

[22] Personal interview with Richard Friedman, MD 12 Apr. 2015.

[23] See Bonnie Bainbridge Cohen's work, Body Mind Centering. 7 Nov. 2016 bodymindcentering.com Also see Mary Overlie's Six Viewpoints theory of movement, 7 Nov. 2016 sixviewpoints.com.

[24] The Hara - Shiatsu and other Natural Health healing techniques. 13 November 2016. http://shiatsuman.com/the_hara.php

[25] Slowiak, James. "'Exercises,' Published in Dialog, N. 12, December 1979. Copyright by Jerzy Grotowski, 1979. Translated from the French and Italian Versions by James Slowiak." pp. 160–161. See also Jerzy Grotowski, Towards a Poor Theatre.

[26] Jerzy Grotowski, Towards a Poor Theatre. 1975. 7 Nov. 2016https://www.amazon.com/Towards-Theatre-Performance-Grotowski-Paperback/dp/B00LLOW6TW/ref=sr_1_4?ie=UTF8&qid=1478456770&sr=8-4&keywords=Towards+a+Poor+Theatre.

[27] Nelson, Valerie. "O. Carl Simonton Dies at 66; Oncologist Pioneered Mind-Body Connection to Fight Cancer" - LA Times. 3 July 2009 23 Oct 2016 http://www.latimes.com/nation/la-me-carl-simonton3-2009jul03-story.html.

[28] Ibid. Nelson, Valerie. "O. Carl Simonton Dies at 66; Oncologist Pioneered Mind-Body Connection to Fight Cancer" - LA Times. 3 July 2009, 23 Oct 2016 http://www.latimes.com/nation/la-me-carl-simonton3-2009jul03-story.html.

[29] Getting Well Again: The Bestselling Classic About the Simontons' Revolutionary Lifesaving Self-Awareness Techniques: O. Carl Simonton M.D., James Creighton Ph.D., Stephanie Matthews Simonton, 9780553280333: Amazon.com: Books.
23 Oct. 2016 https://www.amazon.com/Getting-Well-Again-Bestselling-Revolutionary/dp/0553280333/ref=sr_1_1?ie=UTF8&qid=1477245718&sr=8-1&keywords=simontons.

[30] Personal interview with Steve Cole 16 Mar. 2015.

[31] Crazy Sexy Cancer Tips: Kris Carr, Sheryl Crow: 9781599212319: Amazon.com: Books 23 Oct. 2016 https://www.amazon.com/Crazy-Sexy-Cancer-Tips-Kris/dp/1599212315/ref=sr_1_2?ie=UTF8&qid=1477262944&sr=8-2&keywords=kris+carr+crazy+sexy+cancer.

[32] Defaunation in the Anthropocene | Science. 28 Oct. 2016 http://science.sciencemag.org/content/345/6195/401.

[33] World Wildlife "Falls by 58% in 40 Years" - BBC News 28 Oct. 2016 http://www.bbc.com/news/science-environment-37775622.

[34] Earth Is on Brink of a Sixth Mass Extinction, Scientists Say, and It's Humans' Fault - The Washington Post 28 Oct. 2016 https://www.washingtonpost.com/news/morning-mix/wp/2015/06/22/the-earth-is-on-the-brink-of-a-sixth-mass-extinction-scientists-say-and-its-humans-fault.

[35] E.P.A Says Carbon Tetrachloride Spill in Ohio River, Moving Faster Than Predicted, Is Past Cincinnati - The New York Times 28 Oct. 2016 http://www.nytimes.com/1977/02/20/archives/epa-says-carbon-tetrachloride-spill-in-ohio-river-moving-faster.html?_r=0.

[36] A Reevaluation of Cancer Incidence near the Three Mile Island Nuclear Plant: The Collision of Evidence and Assumptions. 28 Oct. 2016 https://www.ncbi.nlm.nih.gov/pmc/articles/PMC1469835/.

Incidence of Thyroid Cancer in Residents Surrounding the Three Mile Island Nuclear Facility. - PubMed - NCBI 28 Oct. 2016 https://www.ncbi.nlm.nih.gov/pubmed/18300710.

Health Studies | Three Mile Island Alert. 28 Oct. 2016 http://www.tmia.com/taxonomy/term/.

[37] Nearly Completed Nuclear Plant Will Be Converted to Burn Coal 28 Oct. 2016. http://www.nytimes.com/1984/01/22/us/nearly-completed-nuclear-plant-will-be-converted-to-burn-coal.html

[38] Chernobyl | Chernobyl Accident | Chernobyl Disaster - World Nuclear Association 28 Oct. 2016 http://www.world-nuclear.org/information-library/safety-and-security/safety-of-plants/chernobyl-accident.aspx.

[39] Flint Water Crisis: A Step-By-Step Look At What Happened : The Two-Way : NPR 28 Oct. 2016 http://www.npr.org/sections/thetwo-way/2016/04/20/465545378/lead-laced-water-in-flint-a-step-by-step-look-at-the-makings-of-a-crisis.

[40] Death and Extinction of the Bees | Global Research - Centre for Research on Globalization 28 Oct. 2016 http://www.globalresearch.ca/death-and-extinction-of-the-bees/5375684.

[41] Colony Collapse Disorder Is No Longer the Existential Threat to Honeybees You Thought It Was. 28 Oct. 2016 http://www.slate.com/articles/health_and_science/science/2016/07/colony_collapse_disorder_is_no_longer_the_existential_threat_to_honeybees.html.

[42] Radical Remission: Surviving Cancer Against All Odds: Kelly A., PhD Turner: 9780062268747: Amazon.com: Books. 2 Nov. 2016

https://www.amazon.com/Radical-Remission-Surviving-Cancer-Against/dp/0062268740/ref=cm_cr_arp_d_product_top?ie=UTF8.

[43] Personal interview with Minas Chrysopoulo, MD 26 May 2015.

[44] Crazy Sexy Cancer Tips: Kris Carr, Sheryl Crow: 9781599212319: Amazon.com: Books 23 Oct. 2016 https://www.amazon.com/Crazy-Sexy-Cancer-Tips-Kris/dp/1599212315/ref=sr_1_2?ie=UTF8&qid=1477262944&sr=8-2&keywords=kris+carr+crazy+sexy+cancer.

[45] Grace and Grit: Spirituality and Healing in the Life and Death of Treya Killam Wilber: Ken Wilber: 9781570627422: Amazon.com: Books 23 Oct. 2016 https://www.amazon.com/Grace-Grit-Spirituality-Healing-Killam/dp/1570627428/ref=sr_1_1?ie=UTF8&qid=1477258280&sr=8-1&keywords=Grace+and+Grit.

[46] Ibid. Wilber pp. 258-259.

[47] Ibid. Wilber, p. 259.

[48] Wilber, p. 260.

[49] "Cytochrome P450." Wikipedia, 30 Oct. 2016. Wikipedia, https://en.wikipedia.org/w/index.php?title=Cytochrome_P450&oldid=746863378

Cytochrome P450 - Wikipedia. 2 Nov. 2016 https://en.wikipedia.org/wiki/Cytochrome_P450.

[50] Personal interview with Steve Cole, PhD 16 Mar. 2015.

[51] Storr, Will. A Better Kind of Happiness - The New Yorker. 30 Oct. 2016 http://www.newyorker.com/tech/elements/a-better-kind-of-happiness?mbid=social_facebook.

[52] Mukherjee, Siddhartha. The Emperor of All Maladies: A Biography of Cancer. Reprint edition, Scribner, 2011.

[53] New Genetics Discovery Paves the Way to Transform Immunotherapy Treatments 31 Oct. 2016 https://www.ucl.ac.uk/cancer/news/new-landmark-genetics-discovery-paves-the-way-to-transform-immunotherapy-treaments.

[54] Everything You Need to Know About CRISPR, the New Tool That Edits DNA 1 Nov. 2016 http://gizmodo.com/everything-you-need-to-know-about-crispr-the-new-tool-1702114381.

[55] Scientists Announce HGP-Write, Project to Synthesize the Human Genome - The New York Times 1 Nov. 2016 http://www.nytimes.com/2016/06/03/science/human-genome-project-write-synthetic-dna.html?_r=1.

The Genome Project–Write | Science 1 Nov. 2016
http://science.sciencemag.org/content/early/2016/06/01/science.aaf6850.

[56] Environmental Epigenomics and Disease Susceptibility. - PubMed - NCBI. 1 Nov. 2016 https://www.ncbi.nlm.nih.gov/pubmed/17363974.

[57] Epigenetics: Fundamentals | What Is Epigenetics? 1 Nov. 2016 http://www.whatisepigenetics.com/fundamentals/.

[58] BRCA1 and BRCA2 Gene Mutations - Know:BRCA 1 Nov. 2016 https://www.knowbrca.org/Learn/brca1-and-brca2-gene-mutations.

[59] The Ancestor Syndrome: Transgenerational Psychotherapy and the Hidden Links in the Family Tree 1st (First) Edition by Schutzenberger, Anne Ancelin Published by Routledge (1998): Amazon.com: Books 1 Nov. 2016 https://www.amazon.com/Ancestor-Syndrome-Transgenerational-Psychotherapy-Schutzenberger/dp/B00E31KYOO/ref=sr_1_2?s=books&ie=UTF8&qid=1478035566&sr=1-2&keywords=the+ancestor+syndrome.

[60] Rachel Yehuda Discusses How Trauma Can Affect Our DNA – Tablet Magazine 1 Nov. 2016 http://www.tabletmag.com/jewish-arts-and-culture/books/187555/trauma-genes-q-a-rachel-yehuda.

[61] Final Report | Markers of Individual Susceptibility and Outcome Related to Fetal and Infant Growth and Development| Research Project Database | NCER | ORD | US EPA 1 Nov. 2016 https://cfpub.epa.gov/ncer_abstracts/index.cfm/fuseaction/display.highlight/abstract/6130/report/F.

[62] Personal interview with Richard Friedman, MD 12 Apr. 2015.

Bibliography

A Reevaluation of Cancer Incidence near the Three Mile Island Nuclear Plant: The Collision of Evidence and Assumptions. https://www.ncbi.nlm.nih.gov/pmc/articles/PMC1469835/. Accessed 28 Oct. 2016.

"About BRCA1, BRCA2, and Hereditary Breast and Ovarian Cancers." *Know:BRCA,* https://www.knowbrca.org/Provider/FNA/about-brca1-brca2-and-hereditary-breast-and-ovarian-cancers. Accessed 16 July 2016.

Amazon.com: Silent Spring: Books. https://www.amazon.com/s/ref=nb_sb_ss_c_2_13?url=search-alias%3Dstripbooks&field-keywords=silent+spring&sprefix=Silent+Spring%2Caps%2C296&crid=2K60G3S5222X5. Accessed 28 Oct. 2016.

Aposhyan, Susan. *Body-Mind Psychotherapy: Principles, Techniques, and Practical Applications.* W. W. Norton & Company, 2004.

Armstrong, K, et al. "Early Adoption of BRCA1/2 Testing: Who and Why."

   Genet Med, vol. 5, no. 2, Apr. 2003, pp. 92–8,

   http://www.ncbi.nlm.nih.gov/pubmed/12644778.

Asher, MD, Arash. *Personal Interview*. 23 June 2015.

Barbara Brennan School of Healing. http://www.barbarabrennan.com/.

   Accessed 24 July 2016.

Barstis MD, John. *Personal Interview*. 26 Mar. 2015.

Bledy, Chris. *Beating Ovarian Cancer: How To Overcome The Odds And*

   Reclaim Your Life. Book Clearing House, 2008.

"Body Psychotherapy." *Wikipedia, the Free Encyclopedia*, 22 May 2016.

   Wikipedia,

   https://en.wikipedia.org/w/index.php?title=Body_psychotherapy&ol

   did=721507414.

Body-Mind Centering | BMC - An Embodied Approach to Movement, Body

   and Consciousness. http://www.bodymindcentering.com/. Accessed

   6 Nov. 2016.

Books and DVDs | Body-Mind Centering.

   http://www.bodymindcentering.com/store. Accessed 6 Nov. 2016.

"BrainyQuote - Citation." *BrainyQuote*,

   https://www.brainyquote.com/citation/quotes/quotes/v/viktorefr1534

   08.html. Accessed 10 Oct. 2016.

BRCA1 and BRCA2 Gene Mutations - Know:BRCA.

https://www.knowbrca.org/Learn/brca1-and-brca2-gene-mutations.

Accessed 1 Nov. 2016.

Brennan, Barbara. *Hands of Light: A Guide to Healing Through the Human*

Energy Field. Reissue edition, Bantam, 1988.

Chernobyl | Chernobyl Accident | Chernobyl Disaster - World Nuclear

Association. http://www.world-nuclear.org/information-

library/safety-and-security/safety-of-plants/chernobyl-accident.aspx.

Accessed 28 Oct. 2016.

Chrysopoulo, MD, Minas. *Personal Interview.* 26 May 2015.

Cole, PhD, Steve. *Personal Interview.* 16 Mar. 2015.

Colony Collapse Disorder Is No Longer the Existential Threat to Honeybees

You Thought It Was.

http://www.slate.com/articles/health_and_science/science/2016/07/c

olony_collapse_disorder_is_no_longer_the_existential_threat_to_ho

neybees.html. Accessed 28 Oct. 2016.

Crazy Sexy Cancer Survivor: More Rebellion and Fire for Your Healing

Journey: Kris Carr, Marianne Williamson: 9781599213705:

Amazon.com: Books.

https://www.amazon.com/Crazy-Sexy-Cancer-Survivor-

Rebellion/dp/1599213702/ref=sr_1_7?s=books&ie=UTF8&qid=146

6085496&sr=1-7&keywords=kris+carr. Accessed 16 June 2016.

Crazy Sexy Cancer Tips: Kris Carr, Sheryl Crow: 9781599212319:

  Amazon.com: Books. https://www.amazon.com/Crazy-Sexy-Cancer-

  Tips-

  Kris/dp/1599212315/ref=sr_1_2?ie=UTF8&qid=1477262944&sr=8-

  2&keywords=kris+carr+crazy+sexy+cancer. Accessed 23 Oct. 2016.

CROSSING BROOKLYN FERRY. (Leaves of Grass (1860–61)) - The Walt

  Whitman Archive.

  http://www.whitmanarchive.org/published/LG/1860/poems/122.

  Accessed 23 Sept. 2016.

Cshpoemsbywaltwhitman.

  http://www.rainsnow.org/csh_poems_by_walt_whitman.htm.

  Accessed 29 Sept. 2016.

"Cytochrome P450." *Wikipedia*, 30 Oct. 2016. *Wikipedia*,

  https://en.wikipedia.org/w/index.php?title=Cytochrome_P450&oldid

  =746863378.

Cytochrome P450 - Wikipedia.

  https://en.wikipedia.org/wiki/Cytochrome_P450. Accessed 2 Nov.

  2016.

D, Stephen M.Johnson Ph. *Character Styles*. 1 edition, W. W. Norton &

  Company, 1994.

Death and Extinction of the Bees | Global Research - Centre for Research on Globalization. http://www.globalresearch.ca/death-and-extinction-of-the-bees/5375684. Accessed 28 Oct. 2016.

Defaunation in the Anthropocene | Science. http://science.sciencemag.org/content/345/6195/401. Accessed 28 Oct. 2016.

Earth Is on Brink of a Sixth Mass Extinction, Scientists Say, and It's Humans' Fault - The Washington Post. https://www.washingtonpost.com/news/morning-mix/wp/2015/06/22/the-earth-is-on-the-brink-of-a-sixth-mass-extinction-scientists-say-and-its-humans-fault/. Accessed 28 Oct. 2016.

Environmental Epigenomics and Disease Susceptibility. - PubMed - NCBI. https://www.ncbi.nlm.nih.gov/pubmed/17363974. Accessed 1 Nov. 2016.

E.P.A Says Carbon Tetrachloride Spill in Ohio River, Moving Faster Than Predicted, Is Past Cincinnati - The New York Times. http://www.nytimes.com/1977/02/20/archives/epa-says-carbon-tetrachloride-spill-in-ohio-river-moving-faster.html?_r=0. Accessed 28 Oct. 2016.

Epigenetics: Fundamentals | What Is Epigenetics?

    http://www.whatisepigenetics.com/fundamentals/. Accessed 1 Nov.

    2016.

Everything You Need to Know About CRISPR, the New Tool That Edits DNA.

    http://gizmodo.com/everything-you-need-to-know-about-crispr-the-

    new-tool-1702114381. Accessed 1 Nov. 2016.

Final Report | Markers of Individual Susceptibility and Outcome Related to

    Fetal and Infant Growth and Development| Research Project

    Database | NCER | ORD | US EPA.

    https://cfpub.epa.gov/ncer_abstracts/index.cfm/fuseaction/display.hi

    ghlight/abstract/6130/report/F. Accessed 1 Nov. 2016.

Flint Water Crisis: A Step-By-Step Look At What Happened : The Two-Way :

    NPR. http://www.npr.org/sections/thetwo-

    way/2016/04/20/465545378/lead-laced-water-in-flint-a-step-by-step-

    look-at-the-makings-of-a-crisis. Accessed 28 Oct. 2016.

Fox, Susannah, and Lee Rainie. "Part 1: How the Internet Has Woven Itself

    into American Life." *Pew Research Center: Internet, Science &*

    Tech, 27 Feb. 2014, http://www.pewinternet.org/2014/02/27/part-1-

    how-the-internet-has-woven-itself-into-american-life/.

Frankl, Viktor E., et al. *Man's Search for Meaning.* 1 edition, Beacon Press,

    2006.

Friedman, MD, Richard. *Personal Interview.* 12 Apr. 2015.

Getting Well Again: The Bestselling Classic About the Simontons'

Revolutionary Lifesaving Self- Awareness Techniques: O. Carl

Simonton M.D., James Creighton Ph.D., Stephanie Matthews

Simonton, Stephanie Matthews, James L. Creighton:

9780553280333: Amazon.com: Books.

https://www.amazon.com/Getting-Well-Again-Bestselling-

Revolutionary/dp/0553280333/ref=sr_1_1?ie=UTF8&qid=14772457

18&sr=8-1&keywords=simontons. Accessed 23 Oct. 2016.

Grace and Grit: Spirituality and Healing in the Life and Death of Treya

Killam Wilber: Ken Wilber: 9781570627422: Amazon.com: Books.

https://www.amazon.com/Grace-Grit-Spirituality-Healing-

Killam/dp/1570627428/ref=sr_1_1?ie=UTF8&qid=1477258280&sr=

8-1&keywords=Grace+and+Grit. Accessed 23 Oct. 2016.

Grotowski, Jerzy. *Interview with Jerzy Grotowski by James Slowiak.* Dec.

1979. Dialogue N, 12.

Hass, Robert. *Praise.* Ecco, 1999.

Health Studies | Three Mile Island Alert.

http://www.tmia.com/taxonomy/term/12. Accessed 28 Oct. 2016.

"History of Philosophy." *History of Philos,*

https://archive.org/stream/historyofphiloso02wind#page/406/mode/2

up/search/spatiality. Accessed 16 Oct. 2016.

Hoaglund, Tony. *The Hero's Journey.*

Incidence of Thyroid Cancer in Residents Surrounding the Three Mile Island

    Nuclear Facility. - PubMed - NCBI.

    https://www.ncbi.nlm.nih.gov/pubmed/18300710. Accessed 28 Oct.

    2016.

Jeung, In Cheul, et al. "Primary Carcinoma of the Fallopian Tube: Report of

    Two Cases with Literature Review." *Cancer Research and*

    Treatment : Official Journal of Korean Cancer Association, vol. 41,

    no. 2, June 2009, pp. 113–116. *PubMed Central*,

    doi:10.4143/crt.2009.41.2.113.

Kitchen Table Wisdom: Stories That Heal, 10th Anniversary Edition: Rachel

    Naomi Remen: 9781594482090: Amazon.com: Books.

    https://www.amazon.com/Kitchen-Table-Wisdom-Stories-

    Anniversary/dp/1594482098/ref=sr_1_1?ie=UTF8&qid=147726214

    4&sr=8-1&keywords=Naomi+Remen. Accessed 23 Oct. 2016.

Landau, Deborah. "Solitaire." *The Uses of the Body.*

Language of the Body: Alexander Lowen: 9780020773108: Amazon.com:

    Books. https://www.amazon.com/Language-Body-Alexander-

    Lowen/dp/0020773102/ref=sr_1_2?s=books&ie=UTF8&qid=14782

    89056&sr=1-

    2&keywords=alexander+lowen+the+language+of+the+body.

    Accessed 4 Nov. 2016.

Life Over Cancer: The Block Center Program for Integrative Cancer

   Treatment: Keith Block, Andrew Weil M.D.: 9780553801149:

   Amazon.com: Books. https://www.amazon.com/Life-Over-Cancer-

   Integrative-

   Treatment/dp/0553801147/ref=sr_1_1?ie=UTF8&qid=1476656537

   &sr=8-1&keywords=Block+cancer. Accessed 16 Oct. 2016.

Light Emerging: The Journey of Personal Healing: Barbara Brennan:

   9780553354560: Amazon.com: Books.

   https://www.amazon.com/Light-Emerging-Journey-Personal-

   Healing/dp/0553354566/ref=pd_bxgy_14_img_2?ie=UTF8&psc=1&

   refRID=MM1ENG65E66K86BG79SW. Accessed 23 July 2016.

Lorusso, D., et al. "The Role of Secondary Surgery in Recurrent Ovarian

   Cancer." *International Journal of Surgical Oncology*, vol. Volume

   2012 (2012), Article ID 613980, Mar. 2012, p. 6 pages,

   http://www.hindawi.com/journals/ijso/2012/613980/.

Lowen, Alexander. *Language of the Body*. Macmillan General Reference,

   1971.

Lowry, Fran. *Long-Term Survival for Ovarian Cancer Higher Than Thought*.

   http://www.medscape.com/viewarticle/849604. Accessed 18 Sept.

   2016.

Martha: The Life and Work of Martha Graham- A Biography: Agnes De

   Mille: 9780394556437: Amazon.com: Books.

https://www.amazon.com/Martha-Life-Work-Graham-
Biography/dp/0394556437/ref=sr_1_6?ie=UTF8&qid=1478289871
&sr=8-6&keywords=Martha+Graham. Accessed 4 Nov. 2016.

Mille, Agnes De. *Martha: The Life and Work of Martha Graham- A
Biography.* 1st edition, Random House, 1991.

Mukherjee, Siddhartha. *The Emperor of All Maladies: A Biography of
Cancer.* Reprint edition, Scribner, 2011.

The Gene: An Intimate History. 1 edition, Scribner, 2016.

*My Grandfather's Blessings: Stories of Strength, Refuge, and Belonging:
Rachel Naomi Remen: 9781573228565: Amazon.com: Books.*
https://www.amazon.com/My-Grandfathers-Blessings-Strength-
Belonging/dp/1573228567/ref=sr_1_2?ie=UTF8&qid=1477262144
&sr=8-2&keywords=Naomi+Remen. Accessed 23 Oct. 2016.

Nearly Completed Nuclear Plant Will Be Converted to Burn Coal.
http://www.nytimes.com/1984/01/22/us/nearly-completed-nuclear-
plant-will-be-converted-to-burn-coal.html. Accessed 28 Oct. 2016.

Nelson, Valerie. *O. Carl Simonton Dies at 66; Oncologist Pioneered Mind-
Body Connection to Fight Cancer - LA Times.* 3 July 2009,
http://www.latimes.com/nation/la-me-carl-simonton3-2009jul03-
story.html.

*New Genetics Discovery Paves the Way to Transform Immunotherapy
Treatments.* https://www.ucl.ac.uk/cancer/news/new-landmark-

genetics-discovery-paves-the-way-to-transform-immunotherapy-

treaments. Accessed 31 Oct. 2016.

Nye, Naomi Shihab. "Kindness." *"Kindness" from Words Under the Words:*

Selected Poems by Naomi Shihab Nye, Copyright © 1995. Reprinted

with the Permission of Far Corner Books.

Pregnant 9/11 Survivors Transmitted Trauma to Their Children | Science |

The Guardian.

https://www.theguardian.com/science/neurophilosophy/2011/sep/09/

pregnant-911-survivors-transmitted-trauma. Accessed 1 Nov. 2016.

Rachel Yehuda Discusses How Trauma Can Affect Our DNA – Tablet

Magazine. http://www.tabletmag.com/jewish-arts-and-

culture/books/187555/trauma-genes-q-a-rachel-yehuda. Accessed 1

Nov. 2016.

Radical Remission: Surviving Cancer Against All Odds: Kelly A., PhD

Turner: 9780062268747: Amazon.com: Books.

https://www.amazon.com/Radical-Remission-Surviving-Cancer-

Against/dp/0062268740/ref=cm_cr_arp_d_product_top?ie=UTF8.

Accessed 2 Nov. 2016.

Recurrent Epithelial Ovarian Cancer. 15 Apr. 2013,

http://www.cancernetwork.com/oncology-journal/recurrent-

epithelial-ovarian-cancer-update-treatment.

Reductionism and Holism in Psychology | Simply Psychology.

   http://www.simplypsychology.org/reductionism-holism.html.

   Accessed 16 Oct. 2016.

René Descartes - Wikipedia.

   https://en.wikipedia.org/wiki/Ren%C3%A9_Descartes. Accessed 16

   Oct. 2016.

Scientists Announce HGP-Write, Project to Synthesize the Human Genome -

   The New York Times.

   http://www.nytimes.com/2016/06/03/science/human-genome-

   project-write-synthetic-dna.html?_r=1. Accessed 1 Nov. 2016.

Servan-Schreiber, David. *Anticancer: A New Way of Life.* New edition,

   Viking, 2009.

Shepherd, Philip, and Andrew Harvey. *New Self, New World: Recovering*

   Our Senses in the Twenty-First Century. Original edition, North

   Atlantic Books, 2010.

Slowiak, James. "'Exercises,' Published in Dialog, N. 12, December 1979.

   Copyright by Jerzy Grotowski, 1979. Translated from the French

   and Italian Versions by James Slowiak." *Dialog*, vol. No. 12, Dec.

   1979, p. 160–161.

"Stage IV Ovarian Cancer." *CancerConnect News*, 23 Mar. 2004,

   http://news.cancerconnect.com/stage-iv-ovarian-cancer/.

Storr, Will. *A Better Kind of Happiness - The New Yorker*.

http://www.newyorker.com/tech/elements/a-better-kind-of-happiness?mbid=social_facebook. Accessed 30 Oct. 2016.

Survival Rates for Ovarian Cancer, by Stage.

http://www.cancer.org/cancer/ovariancancer/detailedguide/ovarian-cancer-survival-rates. Accessed 17 July 2016.

The Ancestor Syndrome: Transgenerational Psychotherapy and the Hidden Links in the Family Tree 1st (First) Edition by Schutzenberger, Anne Ancelin Published by Routledge (1998): Amazon.com: Books.

https://www.amazon.com/Ancestor-Syndrome-Transgenerational-Psychotherapy-Schutzenberger/dp/B00E31KYOO/ref=sr_1_2?s=books&ie=UTF8&qid=1478035566&sr=1-2&keywords=the+ancestor+syndrome. Accessed 1 Nov. 2016.

The Block Center for Integrative Cancer Treatment.

http://www.blockmd.com/blog/ask-dr-block-chronomodulated-chemotherapy. Accessed 16 Oct. 2016.

The Genome Project–Write | Science.

http://science.sciencemag.org/content/early/2016/06/01/science.aaf6850. Accessed 1 Nov. 2016.

The Hara - Shiatsu and Other Natural Health Healing Techniques.

http://shiatsuman.com/the_hara.php. Accessed 19 Oct. 2016.

"The History of the Internet in a Nutshell." *Six Revisions*, 15 Nov. 2009,

    http://sixrevisions.com/resources/the-history-of-the-internet-in-a-

    nutshell/.

The Six Viewpoints. http://sixviewpoints.com/. Accessed 6 Nov. 2016.

Towards a Poor Theatre (Eyre Methuen Drama Books) (Performance Books)

    by Grotowski, Jerzy (1975) Paperback: Amazon.com: Books.

    https://www.amazon.com/Towards-Theatre-Performance-Grotowski-

    Paperback/dp/B00LLOW6TW/ref=sr_1_4?ie=UTF8&qid=14784567

    70&sr=8-4&keywords=Towards+a+Poor+Theatre. Accessed 6 Nov.

    2016.

Trauma: Our Genetic Inheritance - TEDxAmsterdam.

    http://tedx.amsterdam/2014/08/trauma-can-inherited/. Accessed 1

    Nov. 2016.

Turner, Kelly A., PhD. *Radical Remission: Surviving Cancer Against All*

    Odds. Reprint edition, HarperOne, 2015.

Vanschoubroek, Lieve and Michaela Sieh. *Simonton Method / Mind-Body*

    Interventions / CAM-Cancer. 29 Jan. 2015, http://www.cam-

    cancer.org/The-Summaries/Mind-body-interventions/Simonton-

    Method/(merge).

Webdesignerdepotstaff. *The Evolution of Cell Phone Design Between 1983-*

    2009. http://www.webdesignerdepot.com/2009/05/the-evolution-of-

    cell-phone-design-between-1983-2009/. Accessed 9 July 2016.

"What You Need to Know About 4 Gynecological Cancers." *Health*

Essentials from Cleveland Clinic*, 2 June 2015,

https://health.clevelandclinic.org/2015/06/what-you-need-to-know-

about-4-gynecological-cancers/.

Whitman, Walt. "Crossing Brooklyn Ferry." *Leaves of Grass*.

Leaves of Grass.

Windelband, Wilhelm. *History of Philosophy*. revised ed f 1901. Harper &

Bros f Harper Torchbooks 1958,

https://archive.org/stream/historyofphiloso02wind#page/406/mode/2

up/search/spatiality.

World Wildlife "Falls by 58% in 40 Years" - BBC News.

http://www.bbc.com/news/science-environment-37775622. Accessed

28 Oct. 2016.

INDEX

Made in the USA
Middletown, DE
09 July 2022